Beloved J
I'm so grateful for
you! Blessings +
Much love -
Gretchen

One hill, many voices:
STORIES OF HOPE AND HEALING

DONNA CAMERON and **KRISTEN LEATHERS**

J - You are
such a great,
inspiring part of
this book -
1 Hill 9 Kris Leathers

J -
Thanks for sharing your
story, and for your
generous spirit
Donna Cameron

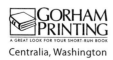

GORHAM
PRINTING
A GREAT LOOK FOR YOUR SHORT-RUN BOOK
Centralia, Washington

Book cover and interior graphic design by Holly Harmon
Back cover and interior photographs by Victrinia Ridgeway
Photo on page 7 by Rodika Tollefson; photo on page 42 by Carolyn McIntyre;
photo on page 202 by Fatema Bannazadeh

ISBN: 978-0-615-51850-3

For inquiries and to order additional copies of this book contact:

Harmony Hill Retreat Center
Union, Washington
www.harmonyhill.org

To all who are seeking wholeness –

with each step, you light the way

for everyone who follows.

CONTENTS

	Prologue	1
Chapter 1	**Finding Our Place, Sharing Our Stories**	5
Chapter 2	**With a Little Help from Our Friends**	22
Chapter 3	**New Beginnings:** *Recovering what was lost*	43
Chapter 4	**Letting Go:** *The gift of vulnerability*	59
Chapter 5	**Dancing with Gratitude**	73
Chapter 6	**Touching Earth, Lifting Spirits**	102
Chapter 7	**Choosing Our Path**	118
Chapter 8	**Tools for the Journey**	136
Chapter 9	**Tears of Transformation:** *Navigating grief and loss*	150
Chapter 10	**Homecoming**	163
Chapter 11	**The Power of Story:** *Where do we go from here?*	180
Appendix I	**Telling Your Story**	190
Appendix II	**Recommended Resources**	192
Appendix III	**Harmony Hill Timeline**	198
	Acknowledgements	201
	About the Authors	202

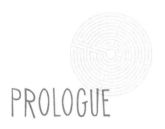

PROLOGUE

I arrive at Harmony Hill out of breath, not the way I'd intended to begin the day at a healing retreat. It's 9:59 a.m., one minute before the program is scheduled to begin, when I park the car. I bound up the brick pathway and burst through the front door of the Great Hall.

People are getting settled in the large circle of chairs in the main room. "Tools for the Journey" is a one-day mini-retreat offered to provide resources and coping strategies to people living with cancer and to their caregivers. It's an abbreviated version of the three-day cancer retreat Harmony Hill is known for. Both are offered at no cost to participants.

There's an ambiguous energy here: expectant, hopeful, and uncertain expressions on the faces of the twenty people gathered here. Some folks are chatting, some flipping through their Cancer Resource notebooks. Others sit in silent anticipation of the day ahead.

The Great Hall's main room is spacious, and although it's a typically drear Pacific Northwest winter's day, the room is warmed by the burnished wood floors and the broad beams overhead; the wall of windows and multiple skylights above draw the soft daylight inside, and a cheerful fire dances in the huge river-rock fireplace. In the center of our circle is a small, low table, bright with fresh flowers and four lit candles.

A dark-haired woman with wide-set eyes and an encouraging smile introduces herself as Kathy – a hospital chaplain, spiritual and grief counselor – one of the two facilitators for the day's retreat. She retrieves from the center table a talking stick, explaining to those who may not be acquainted with the ritual that the stick is to be passed around the circle, and whoever is holding it is the only one allowed to speak. Kathy urges us all to say as much or as little as we feel the need, then she hands the talking stick to her co-facilitator, soft-spoken Melode, who tells us she is a Viniyoga practitioner and teacher before passing the stick to her right.

One by one, we introduce ourselves: the first speaker has an incurable cancer and is here to learn how best to live all the life he has left; he's accompanied by his neighbor who describes her concern for him and her desire to help. Beside the neighbor are a woman who is newly-diagnosed with breast cancer and her supportive friend. The next speaker is tearful and terse, just finished with her round of chemo and radiation. About a third of today's workshop participants are healing practitioners and volunteers; the two women seated to my left are Harmony Hill staff members, who hope to learn how to better serve the community.

Nearly everyone mentions close friends and family members who live with cancer or whose lives were lost to it.

The "Tools for the Journey" workshop varies from the three-day cancer retreats, not just in length, but in that the one-day workshop is not limited to cancer patients only. A few of today's participants are living with other chronic illnesses, such as diabetes. The woman to my right, a health practitioner, describes herself as "probably one of the oldest living survivors of juvenile diabetes." Next, three oncology specialists who have both professional and personal reasons for joining the workshop introduce themselves. One works with the Live Strong Organization, another has initiated an integrative treatment program in the state, and the third admits that she never fully realized what her patients went through until cancer affected her own family.

Seated midway round the circle, Harmony Hill founder and executive director Gretchen Schodde receives the talking stick and explains how Harmony Hill was conceived and developed after she participated in Commonweal's first training for other centers. She also shares that she's had a personal bout with cancer.

"Some of my friends were shocked," she says. "I think they thought that, with the work I do here, I was somehow exempt. I told them I don't think it works like that."

To Gretchen's right is a woman in a wheelchair, swollen and sluggish from medication, who simply tells us her name. Her sister speaks next – about the years of worsening recurrences of cancer and bouts of treatments, the terminal prognosis doctors issued only a day ago. Overwhelmed with the escalating challenges she faces as a caregiver and the prospect of losing her sister, she speaks in a voice tinged with despair. Next, a lively young woman, freshly shaken by her own very recent, unexpected diagnosis, tells us she is determined not to lose her Self to the disease. She passes the stick to a woman who sacrificed both breasts and her uterus in order to survive cancer. Two years later, grateful to have "beat the cancer," she still feels like something is missing in her healing. She says, "It's like the candles inside me were extinguished."

The next speaker grips the talking stick tightly with both hands; she is angry and bewildered at her recent diagnosis; her friend beside her has her own chronic health issues, and they want to help each other persevere. Finally, there is a married couple who've traveled nearly 300 miles to be here; they have grieved the loss of five close family members to cancer within the past year and are now here to help one another cope with the wife's diagnosis of "the family disease."

Once the introductions are completed, we sit in silent contemplation for a few minutes. Then Melode leads us in a breathing exercise. She gently and masterfully guides us through a full-body yawn: a thorough unwinding of every muscle from head to toe, and a total release of all tension. We breathe in healing, we release fear and anxiety, and it feels somehow as if our circle has expanded, as if we have all unfurled.

Next, Kathy outlines the rest of the day's schedule. She then opens a discussion about healing, purpose, and quality of life.

"Today," Gretchen says, "a diagnosis of cancer is not the automatic death sentence it was in the past." With millions of people living with cancer today, cancer is increasingly considered a chronic disease that can be managed. Several survivors in the group note how cancer changes the way you live your life: you figure out what's important, and you learn not to waste your time.

By the end of the discussion, stomachs are rumbling, and it is time for lunch at the Main Lodge. We walk down the short hill in the mist. The fog, thick all morning, still hasn't lifted from the Sound. The dining room itself is elegantly simple and cozy with a fire in the huge fireplace. The sight of the big, farm-style kitchen and the kitchen garden, coupled with the mouth-watering aromas of the foods laid out on the buffet table delights every one of us. We line up and fill our bowls with corn chowder, our plates with savory squash casserole, scalloped potatoes with mushrooms, nasturtium-blessed salad greens, and, for dessert, blackberry crumble.

Breaking bread together in this convivial atmosphere, people begin swapping stories about their travels, their children, their pets. "This is the dog-lovers' table here!" someone declares. There's a rising tenor of camaraderie filling the air by the time I finish my dessert. The hour after lunch is unstructured, so that we may attend the labyrinth orientation, visit the various rooms and buildings, explore the gardens, or just visit with others.

The day is still close and drizzly; the woods are quiet, except for the soft, steady dripping from boughs as I walk the grounds.

It's time to reconvene in the Great Hall for our final ninety minutes together. Behind each chair, a mat, blanket, and pillows have been placed, and Melode invites us all to lie down for a "guided imagery" session. When we are encouraged to invite the spirits of our loved ones and ancestors to join us, I feel the presence of my dear grandmother and my favorite cousin at my side. And then we are being brought back to a reawakened state, to rise, unhurried, and take our seats.

Gretchen has rejoined the group. She guides us through the Cancer Resource notebook – a wealth of information that most of us eagerly annotate. We talk about the challenges of serious illness. We share strategies for talking with our doctors, for dealing with nausea, for sleepless nights. We laugh together over one woman's observation that her cancer appears to be the one thing to finally silence her hypercritical mother-in-law.

 And then it is time to close.

We stand and as I look around the room, it seems to me that in the course of this one, short day, we have all been knitted together, no longer the lone, frayed strangers we were this morning. We take a few deep breaths and then say our goodbyes to one another.

It's dusk. Most of us have a ferry to catch, a couple of hours or more to drive in rush-hour traffic, and so we make our ways to our cars, back to our lives. The heavy fog has lifted from the Sound. In the gloaming, I see a great blue heron perched on a piling. Then another. And another. For miles, on every piling alongside the road, herons are posted like silent sentinels. I feel electric, charged with positive energy, and I can't wait to pass it on. ❧

(K.L.)

CHAPTER ONE:
Finding our place, sharing our stories

"I learned about Harmony Hill from a dear friend whose life was transformed by her retreat there. Before she went, she was bitter, frightened and angry about her diagnosis. But after she returned, she was the most intensely alive person I have ever known, despite the fact that hers was a fairly rapidly terminal disease." – MARJORIE LUCKEY, MD

In its 25-year history, Harmony Hill has touched countless lives, and each of those lives has touched countless others. Harmony Hill is a place of healing, a place of connecting, a place of nurturing, and a place of story. It began as one woman's vision and has grown to be a sanctuary where people whose lives are touched by cancer can go to find physical, emotional, mental, and spiritual healing in a safe and serene setting.

Harmony Hill's mission is to transform the lives of those affected by cancer and to inspire healthy living for all. Three-day and one-day retreats help people dealing with cancer and their caregivers face the challenges of their health issues, activate healing, and restore their quality of life. These are offered at no cost to participants. In addition to its seminal cancer retreats, Harmony Hill offers a wide variety of wellness programs and is also a place for individuals or groups to relax and renew in a breathtaking natural setting.

Harmony Hill is composed of thousands of stories that create and sustain one powerful intention – to heal and to restore wholeness. The power of story is that it may heal and transform teller and listener alike. By sharing stories from the heart – stories about strivings, triumphs and defeats, worries as well as joys – we are reminded that we are all connected, that we matter and that we are not alone.

> **"The world is made up of stories, not atoms."**
> – MURIEL RUKEYSER

At the heart of Harmony Hill is the woman whose compassion, vision and devotion are its foundations. People are drawn to partner in the creation of Harmony Hill because Gretchen Schodde is, as someone once expressed it, "the real deal." She is a source of the "firm persuasion" that William Blake described as "capable of removing mountains." Praise embarrasses her, and she hurries to protest that hers is a small role in the big picture, but one thing cannot be disputed – without Gretchen, there would be no Harmony Hill.

In person, she is an unassuming figure: white-haired, soft-spoken, plainly dressed (often found in galoshes and a floppy rain hat on a typically-wet Pacific Northwestern day.) Hers is a steady presence, yet at the same time she seems to be in constant motion – her keen blue eyes missing nothing, her hands restlessly shuffling papers, taking notes or picking vegetables and deadheading flowers while leading visitors 'round a tour of the Hill. When she speaks, it's often in the nervous, rushed style of someone who doesn't desire the spotlight, but her voice gathers a calm strength as she describes the latest cancer retreat and its participants. This is the life purpose to which she's single-mindedly committed; she's devoted all her estimable energy in service to others.

Literally down-to-earth, she has a passion for gardening that is both a metaphor for her style as executive director and an explanation of her positive outlook. As writer Susan Hill once noted, "The gardener is by definition one who plans for and believes and trusts in the future, whether in the short or the longer term." A healer by nature and by training, Gretchen has an abundant capacity for empathy which has been further honed by her own experience of cancer. She leads by example, and whenever it has looked as if the dream were impossible to realize, her deep connection to a higher spiritual source has endured – and prevailed. If taking great leaps of faith were a marathon sport, Gretchen would have a roomful of gold medals. ❖

GRETCHEN SCHODDE:
FOLLOWING A MOUNTAIN PATH

I was raised on a dairy farm at the base of Mount Rainier. That mountain was the first of many majestic peaks on a path that led me to my ultimate home, to Harmony Hill. In the frequently overcast Pacific Northwest, Rainier is often completely obscured by clouds. We can go for days without seeing it. On a clear day, we say, "The Mountain is out," and its breathtaking presence is a reminder that we may lose sight of our purpose, but it's there, even when hidden from us.

My childhood in the shadow of that mountain gave me so many of the values that have guided my life – love for the soil and for gardening, enjoyment of cooking and healthy foods, a desire to be of service, and trust that the universe supports us when we may not be able to support ourselves. It was there that I first heard the call of medicine and the healing arts.

Initially, I wanted to be a doctor. Today there would be no barriers to that goal, but back then few women were doctors, and those who were needed to be wealthy, to be willing to give themselves to their career, and willing to forsake marriage and a family. At that time, I couldn't check any of these conditions off.

However, I had a misperception about nursing. Nurses, in my experience, worked under the close direction of doctors and were able to exercise little autonomy or independent thinking. I had the great fortune to attend a meeting where a nurse talked about what nurses really do and foretold an exciting new future for the nursing profession: frontier nurses, itinerant public health nurses, nurses who practiced independently and didn't just take orders from doctors. This was a future I could envision for myself; this was a way of practicing patient care that made my heart sing. I enrolled in nursing school and loved every day of it.

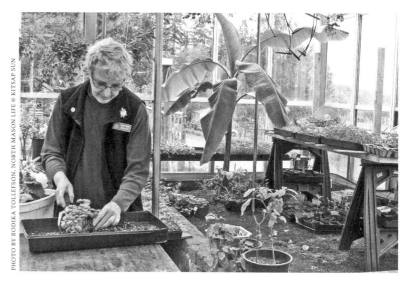

Harmony Hill founder Gretchen Schodde tends to a basil plant inside the spacious greenhouse on the retreat center grounds.

Not long after graduating and becoming a public health nurse, I had an opportunity to go to Bavaria to see where my beloved grandfather was raised. Here, I encountered another mountain that would influence the course of my life. The relatives who picked me up at the train station knew I was not a Catholic, as they were, so out of respect for the beliefs of their cousin from the American West, they replaced the crucifix and rosary beads that usually hung from the rear-view mirror of their station wagon with a picture of Gene Autry. I have vivid memories of the ride up the Alps to their home. As Gene Autry bounced before my eyes, the mountain filled my soul and my late grandfather's presence enveloped me. It was a homecoming and an awakening.

From that village in the high Alps, I took a train to Northern Germany to visit the land where my other grandfather was raised. It was an all-night train ride. I didn't sleep. Throughout the night, the rhythm of the rails danced with the rhythm of my breathing and I was filled with a great sense of peace and deep gratitude. Disembarking from the train the next morning, I had a sudden, clear vision of my calling, to "be part of the creation of an educational, recreational, and therapeutic community."

Returning to Washington, I shared my vision with my father, who felt this was too much for a farm girl from a small town in rural Washington. "What about the cows?" he asked. Despite the clarity of the vision, and the unquestionable call I heard, I also knew that the time was not right. I tucked the calling away, as it turns out, for 15 years.

In the intervening years, another Nurse Practitioner and I served as the sole medical team for the remote community of Darrington, in the foothills of the North Cascades Mountains. Later I joined the faculty of the University of Washington School of Nursing. I loved teaching but was disheartened by the pressures to publish and conduct research that would lead to my Ph.D.

An opportunity to travel to Nepal came up through Johns Hopkins University. It was a medical research expedition. I accepted the opportunity to go, not with any thoughts of enlightenment or spiritual questing in mind, but merely in hopes of pleasing the tenure committee.

Enlightenment – or something like it – came nevertheless. It turned out to be a grueling and dangerous trip, one that challenged my very survival and revealed to me the confusion and despair of the mid-career crisis I was facing. I returned from Nepal acutely aware of how out of balance I was physically, mentally, and spiritually. I felt out of integrity with myself. It was time for a change. I resigned from the University of Washington.

There followed a time of uncertainty and searching, during which I attended a retreat at St. Andrew's Episcopal Retreat Center on a hill overlooking the Hood Canal in Washington's Olympic Peninsula. St. Andrew's looks across the Canal to the Olympic Mountain Range. It reminded me of the mountain in whose shadow I was raised, and of the revelatory mountains of Switzerland. I knew with certainty that I had come home.

I stayed there as a volunteer for a year. There was plenty to do at St. Andrews and in the local community. During that time, I regained my health and got back in touch with my spirit, with the earth, and with the mountains that always seemed to light my path. That long-ago calling which had come to me during a train ride through the Alps reasserted itself, this time saying that the time was right. My spirit soared with the certainty that I was where I belonged and that guidance would surely come to show me what was next. Little did I know that my destiny was right next door, a crumbling property on 11 acres that looked across the Hood Canal to the Olympic Mountain range. Today that view nourishes me daily and it inspires hundreds of people each year to find healing in the midst of life's greatest challenge. ❖

Walking our path, the power of the labyrinth

Some of us know from the first moment of our awareness what and where our place is on this Earth. More often, though, we follow a meandering path that takes us in the direction of our destiny, and just as quickly turns us away from it. The labyrinth is a powerful metaphor for life's winding path.

Harmony Hill has three labyrinths, one designed to accommodate visitors in a wheelchair. Over the years, thousands of people have traversed the labyrinths. Each has taken away something different from the path, and many have left behind them physical or energetic tokens of the experience. ❖

MARIAN SWANSON:
JOURNEY TO THE HEART OF THE LABYRINTH

"This is the stupidest thing I've ever done – I'm just walking in a circle." Those were Marian Swanson's thoughts as Melissa West introduced her to walking the labyrinth at Harmony Hill in the fall of 2000. Marian came to a Harmony Hill cancer retreat on the urging of a friend. She had no pre-conceived notions of what she would find there, merely thinking that a weekend away would probably be a good thing following a year of treatment for breast cancer.

Little did she know how life-changing the weekend would be or how thoroughly the labyrinth would weave its way into her life.

Despite entering the labyrinth with some reluctance and much skepticism, Marian found that by the time she reached the center a change had taken place. "I sat down on the bench in the center of the labyrinth and was overwhelmed by a sense of peace and a feeling of being loved." Within an hour after walking that first labyrinth, Marian was asking herself, "Where shall I build one? How will we build it?"

She bought Melissa's book, *Exploring the Labyrinth*, from Harmony Hill's resource shop and read it through that evening. By the time the retreat weekend was over, the labyrinth "had entered my soul…. I knew after that weekend that I would build a labyrinth somewhere."

"I went home Sunday and web-searched about labyrinths for hours. I barely slept that night, and early the next morning, I wrote a letter to Gretchen, describing to her the call my soul was hearing, and my vision of building a labyrinth in Tacoma for everyone to walk. I especially saw it as part of the healing journey for women with cancer."

Within three months, Marian was part of the Tacoma Labyrinth Project, a dedicated group of strangers who became friends over their shared commitment. After searching many potential sites, they built a beautiful brick labyrinth at Chambers Creek Park in University Place. It is there for anyone in the community to use.

Marian hopes this is just the first of several permanent labyrinths in the Tacoma area – she'd like to see one in a hospital, on the grounds at Fort Lewis, and perhaps in other parks.

She also frequently brings a large canvas labyrinth to churches, schools, and other locations, introducing those interested to the peace and magic of the labyrinth. She has seen first-hand how the simple act of walking the winding path helps people go through grief after a loss, helps them answer deeply personal questions, and helps them to see through new eyes. "The labyrinth is like life: if you keep walking, eventually you'll get to where you're going."

During a labyrinth walk Marian had a powerful vision of her mother walking to join Marian's father and sister, both of whom had died many years before. That same evening, Marian's mother passed away. The vision had prepared her for the loss; it comforted her.

"I almost feel I got cancer to learn about the labyrinth. I was meant to do something with it. That's my gift – to share the labyrinth."

Harmony Hill holds a very special place in Marian's heart. She has referred many people there. "For me it was life-changing. I didn't know it at the time."

"If I get anywhere near Harmony Hill I go back to walk one of the labyrinths. It always feels like coming home. No matter how busy I am, Harmony Hill always reminds me to stop and breathe, and take time for me. I am so grateful for my experience there."

Today, amidst a very busy life and a full-time job teaching special-needs children, Marian still finds time to walk the labyrinth at least a couple of times a month, and she roams a "finger labyrinth" frequently. Sometimes she ponders a question. Other times she simply relaxes into the labyrinth and allows it to provide what she needs.

She's also always on the lookout for places to build or set up labyrinths. "I've made a new friendship out of every one I've worked on."

Someone once told Marian, "You do not choose to work with the labyrinth. The labyrinth chooses to work with you." Marian feels blessed to have been chosen by the labyrinth. "Cancer gave me so much more than it took away." ❖

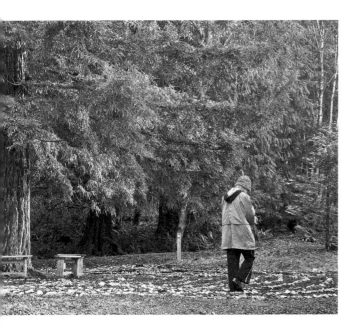

Walking the labyrinth at Harmony Hill.

The labyrinth is an ancient tool for contemplation or meditation. Labyrinths have been traced to 2500 B.C. They are known to have been used in ancient Greece, Rome, and Egypt. The most famous labyrinth is probably the one constructed on the floor of Chartres Cathedral near Paris in about 1220 A.D., still walked by thousands of people each year. Harmony Hill's Redwood Labyrinth uses this classic pattern.

Visitors to the labyrinths at Harmony Hill are encouraged to approach them in whatever way feels right at the time. Some use it as an opportunity to release and relax, to quiet the mind, or simply to be open to whatever they may meet on the path. It is often recommended that the labyrinth be entered with little or no expectation, simply with the willingness to be open to the experience and whatever it may have to offer. Some people formulate a question before entering the labyrinth, then, without conscious effort, find that they receive an answer during the walk or shortly upon completion. Many people find that walking the labyrinth opens them to inspiration, guidance, insight, or understanding.

There are no wrong ways to walk a labyrinth. Walk it in haste, or with slow and measured steps, as a quest, a meditation, or a dance. The intent can be prayerful, curious, open, or whimsical. All the labyrinth asks of us is that we enter it with an open heart and an open mind.

Some labyrinth experts claim that the turns one makes as one walks a labyrinth shifts the awareness from right brain to left brain and back, and that this shifting invites or even induces altered states of consciousness.

The center of the labyrinth is a spot to pause on the bench and enjoy the view; inhale the fragrance of the trees, flowers, and the fresh, invigorating air; listen to the wind rustling in the branches or the sweet harmony of the birds. Many people use a labyrinth's center as a place for meditation or prayer, or simply to enjoy the quiet and receive its gifts. They stay as long as feels right before following the path that leads back out. The "exit" can sometimes bring a sense of empowerment or renewal.

Each time one walks the labyrinth, the experience is different. ❖

MELISSA GAYLE WEST:
SHE WHO NAMES TREES

Psychotherapist Melissa Gayle West encountered Harmony Hill at a time when she wanted a "slow-down" in her therapy practice. She was asked to lead a women's retreat, which was to be on the grounds next door to Harmony Hill.

"During the year we were planning the retreat, Barbara (the woman who was in charge of the retreat) kept trying to get me connected with Gretchen – first of all, because there was a labyrinth over there and we knew we were going to use it for the retreat, and second, because she knew we would just love each other.

"It was a three-day retreat, and on the first evening I was standing outside before dinner and this woman comes to the door, and I just went, 'Oh, my God, I know you!' It was Gretchen. We immediately connected; Barbara was right."

The next day, Melissa took the retreat group to Harmony Hill's redwood labyrinth. She had gotten deeply involved with labyrinths a couple of years earlier. The labyrinth, as she defines it, is "an archetypal map for the healing journey."

"The first time I walked the redwood labyrinth, I showed the women how to do it, and so forth. They started walking it, and I thought, oh, you know, sherry's in about a half hour – this group is Episcopalian, so sherry's at four – I might as well walk it. Why not? So I started walking it and when I got to the redwood and leaned into it, I burst out sobbing. All this grief came up. I was in the process of selling my home, my garden, moving…and I became aware that I hadn't taken the time to honor those losses.

"I just fell in love with that tree. I was so amazed by it that I went home and looked it up – it's a coast redwood. And nobody knows how it got there. It's not native to the area, and there are no other coast redwoods around. Coast redwoods just grow along the coastal region, and the energy they carry is so different than any other tree. For one of the Northern California coast tribes, the coast redwood is considered the wisest of all beings. So I started calling the tree *She Who Knows*; she really is a presence there. I began telling people – as I was orienting them to the labyrinth – that she talks to us. And after that, people started leaving things at the center of the labyrinth at *She Who Knows*.

"Gretchen loves the coast redwood, too, because these trees don't have a deep root system, they have a very shallow one, and the way they're able to support all that weight is that their roots grow with the other redwoods' roots. They support each other. It's very unusual for a tree that size to not have really, really deep roots, but they don't get uprooted because their roots become so entwined with each other that they feed each other. They keep each other upright; they ground each other. And fungi grow which bring nutrients to the tree, and it all becomes a community. Isn't that wild? Talk about intelligent: '*we can't do this by ourselves; we might as well help each other out.*'

"So here's this tree right in the center of Harmony Hill, and Gretchen is like *She Who Knows*, right in the center."

Melissa's involvement with Harmony Hill was an organic process, evolving over the course of ten or twelve years. She had done a lot of teaching and program directing, so it seemed a natural fit when Gretchen asked her to be Harmony Hill's program coordinator. When they got more staff, she became program manager, and when she had even more people under her, she became staff director. She also began to dream with Gretchen what the organization could be, not just in terms of programs, but "bigger and deeper" dreams.

Then in 1999, a, fortuitous thing happened.

"My book agent called and said she had this book she kept thinking that I should be writing, but she had no idea why, and she was quite embarrassed…and she finally said, 'have you ever heard of labyrinths?' Not knowing that I had a 30-foot labyrinth at the house I was then living in, and I was looking out at it as we spoke!

"And so I wrote most of that book [*Exploring the Labyrinth*] at Harmony Hill. It really helped Gretchen get much more into labyrinths, too. There are pictures of Harmony Hill in the book. Gretchen and I used to do tape labyrinths, and she helped me with all the technical stuff in the books. We started dreaming up where different labyrinths could go. We got the lavender one from Evergreen State College. We ordered a canvas one, which we put in the yurt sometimes. Labyrinths were also organic with the growth of Harmony Hill. I used to give labyrinth retreats there, and integrated it into whatever I was teaching, as did other folks on the Hill – it felt like an integral part of what was happening."

Melissa stepped down as program director ("I sort of fired myself") because she was ready to get back to doing more therapy work again. She was then a program consultant from 2006–2007. And always, Harmony Hill remains dear to her.

"There's something special about Harmony Hill that can't be put into words, that has to be experienced. It's a combination of the land, Gretchen, the programs, and the community – not only the staff, but the larger community, as well. There's so much love there and so much caring; the quality of the teaching is so high, and the kitchen, the wonderful food…it's the context there that is greater than the sum of its parts. All come together in a way that helps people experience their wholeness at a deeper level than they ever have.

"I've never experienced a place like that. It really is remarkable. People can go there for any type of retreat, and it's their ticket to that deeper wholeness. *Some people have cancer tickets, some have labyrinth tickets, some people have yoga tickets, some have business retreat tickets…It's an invitation to the whole gestalt.* People are always at a loss to express it, and I think that's because of that synergy. I think it happens at a cellular level for people. You can make cognitive sense of it afterwards. There's something happening at a cellular level or an energetic or spiritual center that is far bigger and deeper than the conscious mind that transforms people.

"My experience in those years that I was at Harmony Hill was not us saying, 'This is what we're going to do,' but rather a deep listening into what was next. And it would always be there, and it was always much bigger than what we thought we could do.

"Gretchen's genius is her ability to hold that much larger space without getting caught in 'the cursed how's.' That's what gets in the way of most people going after their dreams: they get caught up in 'the cursed how's' before they can get energized by the dream. And that will kill a dream faster than anything else. So it's about following a dream and *then* working on 'the cursed how's.'" ❧

> **"**Stories have to repair the damage that illness has done to the ill person's sense of where she is in life, and where she may be going…People tell stories not just to work out their own changing identities, but also to guide others who will follow them. They seek not to provide a map that can guide others – each must create his own – but rather to witness the experience of reconstructing one's own map."
>
> – ARTHUR W. FRANK:
> THE WOUNDED STORYTELLER: BODY, ILLNESS & ETHICS

Garden of earthly delights

Like a pivotal character in a good novel, the gardens at Harmony Hill play an important role in the experience of every visitor. Driving up the steep, winding driveway to the Hill a profusion of lush greenery is the first thing one notices. Depending on the time of year, the sweet fragrance of roses, the calming aroma of lavender, or the spicy perfume of honeysuckle fill the air. Dazzling colors and varieties of flowers surround visitors and adorn vases in all the public areas. The gardens at Harmony Hill are a true labor of love. Strolling the grounds or walking from building to building, every guest is surrounded by nature's splendor and loving intention. ❖

GRETCHEN:
ROOTS

My father was a superb gardener. I grew up watching the bounty he produced from the earth, as well as his intense delight for gardening. I guess that enthusiasm was contagious. I find I need to feel close to the earth and am able to do that each day by working in Harmony Hill's gardens and walking its labyrinths. They ground me as nothing else.

When I first came to this property I felt called to a simpler lifestyle. I had been invited to caretake the vacant house next door to St. Andrews. It was February of 1986 when I moved in. Within a month I had an opportunity to lease the house. After conferring with neighbors and friends who also saw my vision of it as a place for small group retreats and wellness getaways, I signed the lease and we christened it "Harmony House" – a name which conveyed the idea of balance and congruence. It wasn't until 1990 that we changed the name to Harmony Hill, but you can trace the beginnings of the Hill to that cold winter of 1986.

When I first came to the Hill, the gardens were overgrown and the buildings were in disrepair. There had once been an elegant garden but it was long overgrown with blackberries and alder trees. I decided for that first spring and summer to just have a simple carrot patch in front of the big house. The next year I was feeling much stronger and certainly more ambitious. I asked some of the volunteer firemen I worked with to help me get a vegetable garden started. They came out in force with tractors and heavy equipment. We dug and excavated and leveled, and that first year's garden seemed like a bountiful miracle – a taste of abundance yet to come. Each subsequent year, the garden grew larger and flourished before our eyes. In addition to the myriad vegetables, there were multitudes of gorgeous annual spring flowers, such as rhodies, azaleas and daffodils. They inspired us to continue expanding the gardens, enhancing the Hill's grounds, and making the property ever more beautiful. ❖

The gardens have become a character in many people's personal stories. Whether there for a cancer retreat, a wellness workshop, or a few days of personal sanctuary, visitors may carry home with them the peace they experienced sitting by the grape arbor looking across the Hood Canal to the Olympic Mountains. Or perhaps they were able to let go of long-held fears and discover a deep inner knowing as they rested among the fragrant lavender near the Great Hall. ❖

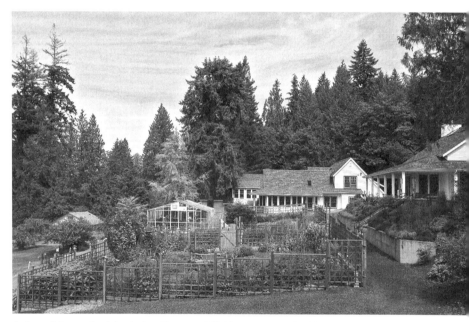

A view of the garden labyrinth at Harmony Hill. Flowers, trees, shrubbery, vegetable and herb gardens, and other well-kept vegetation are in abundance on the campus.

"Everything that slows us down and forces patience, everything that sets us back into the slow circles of nature, is a help. Gardening is an instrument of grace."

– MAY SARTON

SUSAN KLUDAS:
IT ALL STARTED WITH LAVENDER

Lavender drew Susan Kludas to Harmony Hill in 1999. She had just moved from Spokane to Lewis County. Seeking a retreat in her new locale, she was directed by a friend to Harmony Hill's website.

"I signed up for a women's retreat, which had something to do with dedicating the lavender labyrinth. I drove out, parked, and when I slammed the car door, it was like, 'I'm home.'

"The retreat was just out of this world. During my stay, I ran into the facilities person and asked if there was some work that I could come up there and do, and that's how I started."

While Susan spent the majority of her work life as vocational rehabilitation counselor, she has always indulged a lifelong passion for gardening. And Harmony Hill offered her a wealth of opportunities to "play in the dirt."

"So for about six months I came out weekends or sometimes for a day, planting and pruning. I also organized work parties for friends from Lewis County and Shelton. Then came an opening for a weekend facilities person, and I was pleased to get it. I started coming out every Friday through Sunday, doing night-watch, plus I'd do things like hauling wood. Once I transplanted a whole rose garden."

Susan also worked to get people to donate plants. She propagated vines and rhodies donated by local gardeners; she and her husband planted them all. When a Bremerton store had all kinds of surplus bulbs, Susan planted thousands of bulbs in the rain that winter. All that work was worth it because the following spring's bloom was "just breathtaking."

Then in 2004, Susan's husband, Rodney, began having problems driving and with his memory. He was diagnosed with a brain tumor in 2006.

"It became difficult for me to maintain the property we had; I had to cut back on volunteering at Harmony Hill, and we moved to Chehalis in 2006. I was still able to get up to Harmony Hill about quarterly, anyway, until the last two years. Then my husband had to have someone with him 24 hours a day. Walking became so difficult he would not have been safe at the Hill. In the early years, though, he always liked helping out there, too – gardening, remodeling, things like that."

Susan and Rodney attended the one-day "Tools for the Journey" workshop at Harmony Hill together.

"It was the only time Rodney ever talked about his brain tumor. He's not a very eloquent person when speaking about himself, and I guess it was a great deal of help to him. He introduced himself to the group, saying, 'I have a brain tumor, they tell me, and I don't know what to do about it.'"

For Susan, it was "just so good to hear Rod verbalize." And they both benefited greatly from the caring, from all the information provided to them, and from the experience of being there as a family within the healing circle.

"I felt a great deal of support. Making all the decisions for someone I love, that's not a comfortable thing for me. Surgery was one option we were given, but with frontal temporal dementia and brain atrophy, doctors were fearful that surgery would decrease what quality of life he still had. And that was already shortened.

"Someone made the suggestion that I develop a 'support committee.' I selected two people whom I love but who are less emotionally involved in Rod's physical care. One is a nurse practitioner, who is especially helpful when I have questions about medical procedures."

When she has big decisions to make, such as whether or not Rodney should be placed in care outside of home, she talks it over with her team.

"It's still scary for me, but I don't feel like I'm in isolation making these choices for his life. For me, that's probably the most valuable tool I got from the workshop. But you also can't sell short just the joy of being at Harmony Hill, seeing other people in more difficult situations, and learning to take one minute at time. It bolstered my spirits."

When her friend the nurse practitioner had become exhausted in her own practice, Susan went with her to a "Caring for the Caregiver" retreat at the Hill. It was a chance for Susan to step out of her role as her husband's caretaker to be there for her "wondrous," caregiving friend.

More recently, Susan booked a retreat for about 35 of her church members, ages 2 to 90. In response to the group's requests, there was African and Native American drumming, tai chi, morning stretch and yoga, meditation, and healing. There were activities for children and their parents in the cottage.

"And it was the most glorious thing I have ever seen. They were all so enraptured; they wanted to have a retreat every month!

"All these people have family, and in every family they have someone who has a connection with cancer, and when they know the place and can talk about it, and can say, 'I've been there, I'll show you,' then this loved one can take advantage of the situation and not have to come feeling like a stranger….that's what's exciting to me.

"What makes Harmony Hill so special is the people who work there. I believe the site itself is sacred, and the reason is because of the people who have consecrated it." ❖

"The soul cannot
thrive in the absence
of a garden."

– THOMAS MOORE

Nourishing the body and the spirit: Harmony Hill's kitchen

Nearly everyone who visits Harmony Hill returns home with stories about the "amazing" food they enjoyed there. Harmony Hill has made an art of preparing and serving healthy, organic, and delicious foods, mostly vegetarian. Even the most committed carnivores have expressed delight in the variety and quality of the meals. Many were surprised to realize they hadn't even noticed the meals were meatless. Early on, there were so many requests for recipes of the meals served at the Hill it became evident that Harmony Hill needed to produce a cookbook. Thus far, there have been four editions of the Harmony Hill cookbook, and new recipes are developed all the time. ❖

GRETCHEN:
FOOD FOR THE SPIRIT

As much as I love the garden, I love the kitchen at Harmony Hill equally. I was barely walking when my mother and grandmother started teaching me to cook. I like to think that their remarkable culinary abilities were passed to me as easily as we passed salt or swapped stories in that kitchen that looked out onto Mount Rainier.

Soon after Harmony House was born, I met Elaine Cook, a neighbor whose reputation preceded her. A retired sociology professor, prolific reader, world traveler, gardener, and gourmet cook, Elaine chose Harmony House as a means to enhance her pursuit of wellness. She helped us establish our first kitchen, provided healthful and scrumptious recipes, and even wrote our first cookbook. Elaine was a woman of wit and wisdom and I was thrilled that she agreed to serve on our very first Board of Directors.

In those early years, one of the ways we raised much-needed funds was by renting Harmony House to outside groups for retreats and such. I remember being contacted by one group that was very interested in renting our space, but they required a written statement from our Board describing our stand on religion. I explained to them that Harmony House was an educational organization committed to wellness and personal wellbeing; we took no stand on religion. Well, that was not an acceptable answer and they asked me to bring their request to the Board. When I did that, Elaine indignantly declared, "That is religious urinalysis!" Then she said, "Gretchen, your job is to tell them – politely – to go to hell!" I don't remember exactly what I said to them, but they sure didn't hold their retreat at Harmony House! I learned a lot from Elaine's blunt good sense!

Elaine's belief in our vision, her guidance and support, were inspiring to us then, and remain so today, long after she is gone. It was she who insisted to the Board that we must expand the kitchen. Even though we didn't have funds to do so at the time, she saw it as essential to our growth and our success. Elaine didn't live to see the new kitchen, but when it was completed in 1993, we gave it the name "Cook's Kitchen" in her honor. To this day, I feel her spirit there. ❖

Gretchen recognized the importance of feeding people well. From her experience growing up on a large dairy farm, as well as her year of volunteering at St. Andrew's, she learned: "If you want them to leave with good memories and to come back, you must offer meals and snacks that delight the senses."

Harmony Hill's kitchen virtuosos create such fragrant and colorful meals that guests have been known to take photographs of the buffet! In the early years, Gretchen did most of the cooking. Later she was occasionally helped by part-time workers or board members who had a flair in the kitchen.

Meals can be challenging for those who are dealing with a cancer diagnosis. The effects of chemo, radiation, and other treatments can upset digestion, impede appetite or alter one's ability to taste or swallow. The cooks at Harmony Hill, in consultation with nutritional and medical experts, are accustomed to working with special dietary restrictions or creating new menus to help those for whom food has become a challenge.

The kitchen provides thousands of nutritious and delicious meals each year, using fresh, whole ingredients, locally grown whenever possible. Harmony Hill's kitchen staff – from the cooks to the servers – see themselves as an integral part of the Hill experience. They approach the work they do with loving intention, conscious of the important role healthy food plays in treatment and wellness. And they cherish the privilege of nourishing both the body and spirit of every guest who visits the Hill. ❖

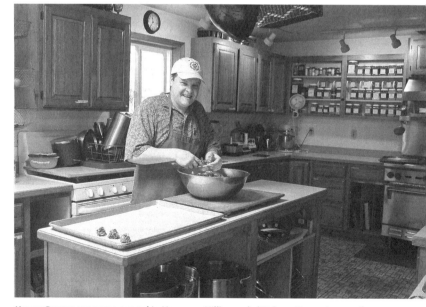

Kenny Brown prepares a meal in Harmony Hill's ample kitchen. Kenny is one of several cooks who prepare the healthy, yet mouth-watering, meals for guests.

CATHY ROGERS:
WHAT WE BRING...

Cathy Rogers, ND, first learned about Harmony Hill during a visit with Michael Lerner at Commonweal in Bolinas, California. Harmony Hill's cancer retreat program was modeled after the groundbreaking program developed there by Dr. Lerner and Rachel Naomi Remen, MD.

She was surprised to learn that there was a place in Washington doing the same kind of work, and that it was on the Hood Canal, just a short distance from her South Sound naturopathy and psychotherapy practice. Cathy was at work on a plan to create a healing center. When she connected with Gretchen some time later, she was delighted to discover that their visions and values as health practitioners were in alignment. They both were committed to wellness, self-care, and to helping people find support and their own inner resources for healing.

Soon after, Cathy joined the faculty at Harmony Hill, first providing classes in nutrition and then facilitating cancer retreats and retreats for caregivers.

At one retreat, Cathy encountered a woman she had known in 7th grade, and hadn't seen for many years. Judy was in the late stages of brain cancer. At the time she and her husband attended the retreat, Judy was unable to eat and was exhausted by her struggles with food and her inability to keep anything down. Cathy's skill as a naturopathic physician and nutrition expert, combined with the superb know-how of the Harmony Hill kitchen staff, created a weekend of meals for Judy that she was able to eat. She immediately experienced a renewal of strength and energy. Judy left with an eating plan that changed her life during her final six months. She was able to eat again, and had the vitality to re-engage with her life, to entertain friends, and to live more fully and normally.

"These things happen at Harmony Hill. Magic happens!" says Cathy.

Cathy sees magic at the retreats for caregivers, as well: "It's easy for caregivers to feel invisible as attention is focused so fully on the person with cancer. When they come to the caregiver retreat, they're acknowledged for what they're going through. They receive some attention, as well as respite, renewal, and a toolbox of skills they can use for their own self-care as they continue the caregiving journey."

During a caregiver session at one cancer retreat, Cathy recalls the breakthrough moment for one individual: "He was the husband of a woman fighting cancer. At one point, he said, 'I'm an engineer; I know how to fix things, and I can't fix this.' That moment of realization lightened his load. His wife was not a 'cancer victim,' and he was not her 'rescuer'; it wasn't up to him to solve this problem like he solved problems in his job. He simply needed to be there for her. It was a moment of profound acceptance and surrender."

It's a lesson Cathy has learned, as well. "As a therapist, you believe you can fix things. But that's not why I'm here. I may have a lot of knowledge and skills, but the most valuable thing I bring to Harmony Hill retreats is just being myself, just being real. I've learned to walk the line between my empathy and having the courage to confront a truth that may be hiding. Or push against resistance if that's what's needed in the moment. Sometimes it's my role to listen and be supportive; sometimes it's my job to name the elephant in the room."

Cathy notes that the two or three retreats she facilitates each year are always inspiring for her. "When people are on the edge of what they believe they can tolerate, it's a pretty potent experience. I'm always reminded of the importance of living in the moment. I'm always put in touch with my own aliveness as I watch people coming up against something that asks so much of them and see them doing the best they can in the face of it. It's easy for all of us to lose touch with what's really important.

"For so long, our culture discouraged talking about illness, especially cancer. We kept hidden what it was like to go through treatment. That's finally starting to change, and, thankfully, Harmony Hill is at the forefront. This is a safe place to talk about cancer, even to joke about it. We talk about the experience of having cancer, the long-term effects and after-effects of treatment. We talk about what the 'new normal' is going to be, and through being so challenged, there is a sense of aliveness that we all feel. Superficialities fall by the wayside.

"Whenever I come to Harmony Hill, I feel in touch with the largeness of life. It's the energetics of the place, the physical environment of the mountains, the water, the gardens, and the spirit of the people who have passed through here – the retreat participants, the faculty, the staff – there is a sacred sense of people's lives being acknowledged here." ❧

Witness

Sometimes the mountain
is hidden from me in veils
of cloud, sometimes
I am hidden from the mountain
in veils of inattention, apathy, fatigue,
when I forget or refuse to go
down to the shore or a few yards
up the road, on a clear day,
to reconfirm
that witnessing presence.

– DENISE LEVERTOV (SELECTED POEMS)

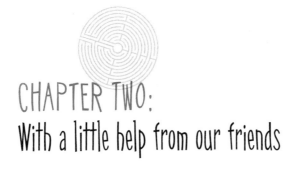

CHAPTER TWO:
With a little help from our friends

"When I was diagnosed with cancer I realized that, while I did not have a choice about the diagnosis, I did have a choice about how I responded. The irony of cancer is that it can provide important gifts and life lessons, even as it threatens life itself. I learned the power of asking for and accepting help – and the gift it provided to others to offer their help and loving support."
– MARIAN SVINTH, 2001 HARMONY HILL ALUMNA

Harmony Hill has been blessed many times by the appearance of friends and supporters at just the moment when most needed: the initial offer to Gretchen to caretake the property in 1986; the purchase of the property by Elmer and Kitty Nordstrom and its subsequent 40-year, rent-free lease to Harmony Hill; seed money and coaching by Bill Gates, Sr., which led to successful fundraising efforts and major program and campus expansions. The Hill has countless friends to whom it is grateful.

Similarly, while traveling a cancer path, many people find it filled with friends along the way – old friends and new ones, and people we thought were just acquaintances, who step forward to ease the burden. Sometimes it's a casserole, or a ride to a medical appointment; sometimes it's a kind word, or a note, or a silent touch that speaks volumes. And sometimes cancer allows us to be the friend we never had time or inclination to be before our diagnosis.

Harmony Hill Cancer Retreat alumni often shake their heads in wonderment at the "gifts" cancer brought them. Said one attendee, "Given a choice, I would never have chosen cancer, but I can't deny how many good things cancer has brought to my life – new priorities, new ways of looking at my life, and, most of all, deeper and truer friendships." ❖

MARION ROY:
THE LIVES WE TOUCH,
THE PEOPLE WHO TOUCH OUR LIVES...

When Marion Roy was diagnosed with late-stage ovarian cancer, she chose to view her illness as a spiritual journey. Marion's daughter, Pam, shared much of that journey with her and describes her mom as having gone through a transformation during that time. "She became a radiant being. It was amazing."

Early in 1996, Marion and her husband, Paul, attended a five-day cancer retreat at Harmony Hill. Despite Marion's acceptance of her diagnosis, it was a desperate time for them, between the weight of treatment and the progression of the cancer. Harmony Hill turned out to be the right place at the right time, and the experience gave Marion a lightness of spirit that remained with her for the months she had left.

"At Harmony Hill, Mom connected with something more powerful than illness. Those five days solidified her transformation and paved more of the spiritual path before her," says Pam.

"It meant so much to her – to both of my parents – to meet others who were going through similar experiences. They were touched by other people's stories and by the genuine love and concern everyone shared. It helped them to feel they were not in this alone. Mom made some deep connections with other retreat participants, connections that lasted until the end of her life."

Both Marion and Paul returned from the retreat deeply moved by the sharing they had experienced and feeling supported by so many people who just days earlier had been strangers to them. Marion's love and concern for the people she had met gave her renewed strength and vitality. Some of the people from the Harmony Hill retreat came long distances to attend the celebration of life held for Marion after her death. One individual wrote Pam expressing how blessed she felt to have known Marion and to have been guided by her wisdom.

A passionate gardener, Marion was also a rock-hound. For many years, she had been collecting rocks on all her travels. Her lovely garden was filled with them. Many were connected to stories of adventure or family outings; they were clustered in places of honor. The rocks gave Marion and her garden a deep sense of calm. Marion was so moved by her experience at Harmony Hill that she wanted her rocks to live on in a new home there after she was gone, and to offer others the same joy and serenity they had given her. Pam remembers driving to Harmony Hill with many buckets of rocks that later graced the perimeter of the tree labyrinth.

"These rocks meant so much to Marion," Gretchen recalls. "To receive them meant as much to us, and they bring to the labyrinth and the people who walk it the same calm and beauty they brought to her. We have been blessed by her gift."

Pam Roy saw the impact of her parents' experience at Harmony Hill. She cherishes the memory of the last months she shared with her mother – rich days, warmed by a radiant wonder. Marion left her daughter some of her mementoes of Harmony Hill: a paper "treasure box" filled with keepsakes from the retreat – moss from the surrounding woods, colorful ribbons, a name badge, a balloon from the closing night celebration, and messages to special people in her life.

"Mom got such a kick out of making this – to her it represented her own vivid and gleaming joyful life. And now I treasure it."

Pam also treasures a letter her mother sent not long before she died. In it, Marion wrote that "the incredible outcome of my cancer is that I have never been happier." She noted that it brought her family closer and she felt "surrounded by more love than I have ever experienced; I am able to give more love to others. I feel freed from the bonds of duty to do all the things I enjoy … new and wonderful people have come into my life, people I never would have met without the cancer."

Through her cancer and her time at Harmony Hill, Marion experienced a profound transformation and deep joy. Her daughter Pam marvels, "It was quite extraordinary. She allowed the fullness of who she was to be wholly expressed. She held nothing back."

Countless Harmony Hill guests and retreat participants have walked the labyrinth and appreciated the beautiful rocks that adorn it. Many have been moved to leave tokens of their own. All are walking in the footsteps of radiant and generous spirits such as Marion Roy. May each of us also follow in Marion's footsteps by allowing the fullness of who we are to flourish…. ❧

GRETCHEN:
FRIENDS INDEED

During that year I stayed at St. Andrew's I found myself settling into the land and surrendering to my life in a way that felt almost pre-ordained. Returning to the basics – the earth, the land, the water – it felt like I was returning to myself. When the opportunity to become caretaker of the property next door arose, I was ready. It was 1986. The property had belonged to the Callison family for many years. When Mrs. Callison died, her family put it up for sale and locals worried that the property would be broken into parcels or sold to be a mobile home park. In exchange for caretaking the large, nearly empty house, I paid rent of $50 a month. Shortly after I settled in and felt my roots starting to take hold, the owners asked me to find someone who would lease the house for a year or more, a difficult task given that the property was for sale.

I knew I wanted to lease the property, but I couldn't be certain that the wellness center I envisioned would thrive in this small community. I needn't have worried. Neighbors were not only supportive, they contributed countless ideas and hours to make the dream a reality. Retired professor Elaine Cook, who lived just down the road, enthusiastically jumped in to help with the garden and the kitchen and, ultimately, joined our Board of Directors. She and neighbor Jean Moore reviewed my grant applications and early marketing pieces and critiqued them with the candor and gentleness of guardian angels. What a lesson in guidance I learned early on from these remarkable and gracious ladies!

If I had any doubts, they were put to rest after talking with Andy Bell, a good friend of my neighbor Gail Forrey. Andy, a quadriplegic since a diving accident when he was in college, was committed to wellness. He saw the house as a place for small group retreats and getaways for himself and others in wheelchairs. He expressed his commitment to "Harmony House," as we originally called it – a place of congruence and wellness. We went to work on the house and on the plans for the organization. Andy later agreed to chair the first board of directors for Harmony House.

In 1988, I received a letter from the Callison's attorney informing me that the property had been sold. The purchasers were Kitty and Elmer Nordstrom. The Nordstrom family had long owned property in Union to which the whole family retreated for vacations and special occasions. Mrs. Nordstrom purchased the property to preserve the land and assure that future generations of her family would always find a peaceful place when they came to their summer homes on the Hood Canal.

I had no idea what this new circumstance would mean for Harmony House. I sat down and wrote a detailed letter to Mr. and Mrs. Nordstrom, describing my dreams for the House. Before mailing it, I asked Jean and Elaine to review the two-page, single-spaced letter. With trepidation, I put in in the mail and waited. As weeks turned to months and there was no response, I started to wonder if I should have written such a long letter to my new "landlords"!

It was a couple of months later, just as I was leaving for work one morning, that I answered the phone to hear, "This is Mr. Nordstrom. Mrs. Nordstrom and I will be out this morning and would like to meet with you." I called Tacoma Community College, where I was teaching, and told them there was no way I could come to work today. A cluster of nerves, I went out and picked a huge bouquet of flowers for Mrs. Nordstrom, and then I baked bread, thinking the fragrance of the bread would be a welcome conversation starter. I invited my neighbor, Gail Forrey, over to join me when the Nordstroms came. Gail knew Kitty, and the two of them chatted in a corner of the living room, while Mr. Nordstrom and I sat by the window.

His legendary business prowess was evident as he patiently and thoroughly grilled me. Who was our attorney? Who was our fiscal agent? How did we plan to raise money? Had we secured our 501(c)(3) tax exemption from the IRS? When did we think we would get it? What exactly where our plans for the House?

They left that afternoon with fresh flowers and freshly-baked bread. Mr. Nordstrom said he wanted to meet with me again when we had received our tax exemption, adding that if we had any troubles with it I should call him because he had someone at the store who was both a CPA and an attorney and could surely help us.

I made arrangements a few weeks later to meet with the Nordstroms again, and Harmony House Board president Andy Bell was going to accompany me. Just as we were getting ready to leave for the meeting, my beeper went off. I had joined the Union volunteer fire department, and was often the only medical professional to respond to aid calls, which this was. I sent Andy on alone to meet with the Nordstroms, hoping I would be able to join him shortly, but it turned out to be a near-fatal accident – a wood-cutter felled by a tree instead of the other way around. I stabilized the bleeding man and went with him to the hospital, where I stayed with him until his family arrived. The ambulance brought me back to Harmony House, just in time to answer another emergency call, another bad one. I didn't get home until late in the evening and fell into bed exhausted, praying there would be no more beeps that night.

I was just waking up at about 7:30 the next morning when I heard knocking at the front door. It was Elmer Nordstrom, checking to make sure I was okay. He also wanted me to take his truck and drive it to Swedish Hospital in Seattle – to which he was closely connected – to pick up a hospital bed and anything else we might need. If Andy or his friends were going to stay at Harmony House, they would need a hospital bed. He would call the CEO of Swedish to arrange for anything we needed. It was clear that Andy had made an impression on them the day before!

I told him I needed to think about what we needed and who I could get to come with me. In truth, I was apprehensive about driving his truck all the way to Seattle. Elmer didn't let me wait him out, though. He kept calling. The supplies were waiting, and he wasn't worried about his truck. I finally summoned my courage and borrowed the truck for the long drive to Swedish Hospital in Seattle. When I got there, I was stunned to find the hospital CEO waiting for me at the loading dock.

They loaded the truck with a hospital bed and other equipment and supplies and I headed back to Union, still dazed by the Nordstroms' generosity. Back at Harmony House, it took a small army of neighbors to unload the truck and transport the hospital bed into the house. We had to take it apart to get it through the front door!

From that point on, Kitty Nordstrom took a great interest in Harmony House, an interest that continued until her death in 2000. She was concerned about the energy it took for me to go out on so many ambulance calls with the volunteer fire department. We shared stories, and she told me about accompanying her father, Dr. Nils Johansen, on medical rounds when she was a young girl. Dr. Johansen was the founder of Swedish Hospital.

The first time she came to Harmony House to have lunch with me, Kitty brought me one of her favorite books, *The Singing Creek Where the Willows Grow*. I had heard that whenever she found a book she liked she bought 10 or 15 copies and gave them to all her friends. A few days after our lunch together she sent me a thank-you gift – a dishwasher. She said I wouldn't have time to be washing dishes with all the people who would be coming to Harmony House! ❖

Early on, Elmer Nordstrom gave Gretchen some blunt advice: "Your board is no damn good unless they know how to raise the money you need to make this work." Gretchen and Harmony Hill boards have taken that guidance to heart, and over the years the Board of Directors has been instrumental in raising funds to meet the mission and finance Harmony Hill's steady growth.

Funds have been raised through direct mail campaigns, auctions, memorial bequests, grants, countless personal donations, product sales, and numerous other creative efforts. Members of the Board see their role as both "making the ask" and coming up with creative ways to attract money to the Hill.

Joan Brekke joined the Harmony Hill Board of Directors eager to help move the Hill ever closer to its mission and vision, but convinced that fundraising was not an activity she would get involved in. "When I was invited to join the Board, I told them that I had no experience in fundraising – and no desire to do it. But I've found that raising money for Harmony Hill is a joyful experience. When people understand what Harmony Hill does, what it means to the people who attend cancer retreats and how their lives are enriched, they open their wallets and their hearts." ❖

One brick at a time

One of the many creative fundraising ideas to emerge in recent years was the creation of a Harmony Hill Tribute Garden Path. The path is paved with bricks that are inscribed with names, memorial messages, celebration announcements, brief love letters, and sometimes inscrutable phrases, the meaning of which may be unclear to all but the purchaser. The bricks come in two sizes – 4" x 8" and 8" x 8" – and can be inscribed with two or three lines of text respectively. Purchased for $100 or $500, they are a forever-link to Harmony Hill and the loved one, celebration, or sentiment inscribed on it.

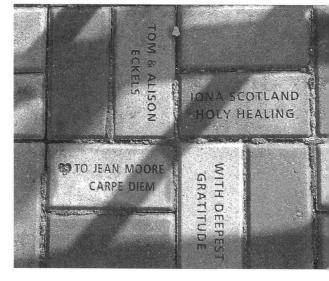

A favorite pastime of visitors is to wander the Tribute Garden, enjoying the fragrance and colors of the many flowers adorning it, while reading the many poignant messages left for posterity. Once the Tribute Path is filled, no doubt other paths will be created to allow people and organizations to celebrate lives and milestones in this warm and welcoming fashion. ❖

JEAN MOORE:
NEIGHBORS TO COUNT ON

Jean Moore has been Harmony Hill's closest neighbor since before it was Harmony Hill, and a friend to Gretchen Schodde for more than 25 years. Jean and her smiling black dog, Lily, hike together daily, passing through Harmony Hill. In her bright yellow shirt and parka, Jean looks like walking sunshine; her blue eyes are keen and merry. A lifelong resident of Hood Canal, 87-year-old Jean is a wealth of local history.

She grew up in Bremerton on the beach. As a young woman, she married, had one child, then divorced and went back to university in Seattle to complete her teaching degree. Around that same time, Jean's mother, also recently divorced, bought the Shelton newspaper from her ex-husband and moved to a little house on the Hood Canal beach. Jean and her son often came out and visited her.

"Little Mike thought it was heaven." Jean recalls. "And I wanted to come back here to live – being on the beach was home. After Mother built the house next to St. Andrew's, I did move here and began teaching. I stayed, and have been here, forever, in that same house."

Jean reminisces about Harmony Hill: "I used to come over here when it was the Callisons' place. The Callison kids grew up here. Their father was a doctor in Seattle, and they spent their summers here. A lot of love has gone into this location, a lot of love for the land. There's something magical in the land itself. I'm not a gardener, but I love it; I like the woods and the beach, that part. For Gretchen, it's the garden. She was a volunteer on the grounds of St. Andrews next door when I first met her.

"Elaine Cook – a professor and a mentor to me and everyone whose life she touched – she saw something special in Gretchen the first time she laid eyes on her. And when she saw something in someone, I really paid attention."

When Harmony Hill started offering the cancer retreats at no cost to participants, Jean was skeptical.

"Elaine Cook, she understood at first; I didn't. I thought it was crazy, this free stuff. How could it possibly be supported? I'm pretty matter-of-fact. But very slowly, it fell into place, the two uses of the place – the paid personal retreats, and the no-cost cancer retreats."

When she was diagnosed with breast cancer, Jean found out firsthand how well Gretchen's vision had been realized.

"Cancer is bad, and it bothered me, but I was over 60 years old, I'd had a good life, I'd been healthy all my life, I had a grown son who was there for me. And I just wasn't afraid. Then I came here, to a Harmony Hill retreat, and I had a wonderful, amazing time.

"I was facing surgery. Women from a church in Tacoma, all of whom had been here before, were here again in my group. They had terrible, terrible cases of cancer. I remember one girl, especially, with young children…so much sicker than I was. And that was the hard part for so many: that they needed to take care of family…a husband, kids. I was scared for the women in my group, not for myself.

"It was a two-day workshop, and I learned a whole lot about the illness in those two days, more than I ever learned from the doctors or anything else. It was a remarkable experience for me, sold me on the whole retreat thing. That's when I began to see how it works. That's when I understood that these women can't pay whatever it would cost to get that kind of care and attention…and whatever that special thing is that Gretchen has.

"Now I just live next door, so I'm here every day. I have Gretchen's attention when I have to have it, which is at least once a week, for anything I want to talk with her about."

Jean is also at Harmony Hill once a week for a meeting of a group she co-founded, the FIEs – the Fiercely Independent Elders.

"When I stopped teaching at 60, I was dying to do things. I started the local chapter of the League of Women Voters. And then four of us – Elaine, myself, Pat and Ray Hanson – started FIE a couple of years after I retired. Everyone lived close. We all loved our homes, and we all wanted to stay in our own homes, too, as we got older. Everybody thought it was a great idea, to form a group like this, but we couldn't find anyone who had done it. Gretchen has been a lot of help, and generous. We went to her in the beginning; we studied it for a year and a half with the help of social workers. We had fun doing it, too, with elegant luncheons, and wine. It's really worked out very well for us. We've made it, and we've supported each other. Some are gone now, but I know that the FIEs helped them.

"FIE is a great experiment. If we didn't have our sense of humor, now, it would be something else again. It gets more ridiculous every year, the older we get. You just have to ride with the laughs. It can be tough; I don't mean to say it isn't. But *the group makes it easier and it makes it joyous.*" ✿

> "A friend is someone who knows the song in your heart, and can sing it back to you when you have forgotten the words."
>
> – DONNA ROBERTS

GRETCHEN:
EXTRAORDINARY GENEROSITY

Once Elmer Nordstrom began to really understand what we were trying to do at Harmony House, his support for our mission extended beyond anything I could have dreamed. In 1990, he and Kitty gave us a ten-year, rent-free lease on the property. Our responsibility was to steward the land and the buildings, and to fund any upgrades. He continually introduced me to his friends and urged them to get involved through funding support or participating in an advisory board he created to counsel us.

I accompanied him once in his truck to pick up a huge fuchsia for Kitty. On our way back, I was driving and my fire beeper went off. It was the middle of the day and there seemed to be no responses to the call. He asked me what it meant. I told him there was a fire near the Alderbrook Golf Course and I should probably get to the fire station to see if anyone had responded. He said, "Gun it!" and we took off through the bumpy logging roads. When we got to the station, no one else had responded so I jumped out of Elmer's truck, grabbed some fire gear and climbed in the smallest fire truck (the only one I could drive). I yelled to Elmer that I'd see him back at his place, then I headed up toward the golf course as fast as I could with the siren blaring. A moment later I looked in my rear-view mirror and saw Elmer right behind me in his truck. The fire turned out to be a fairly small one and shortly after I arrived a few other volunteer firefighters showed up. We put the fire out in short order, with Elmer directing traffic the whole time. He was already in his 80s, but I had no doubt that had he been a few years younger, he'd be signing up for the fire department. I know he delighted in telling Kitty about the joy ride we took her fuchsia on!

My favorite story of Elmer is another one concerning a truck. The little truck I had when we started Harmony House had given up the ghost after a trip over the mountains and I needed to find a replacement. Elmer insisted I borrow his so I could continue to go out on fire calls, but we agreed that I needed to find a good used truck. One Saturday, he offered to accompany me truck shopping. We spent the day tramping through one used car lot after another, finding nothing that would do. Elmer was appalled by the steep prices on beat-up trucks with high mileage. We returned home at the end of a long day no closer to finding a truck and discouraged by the limited choices available to us.

A week later, Elmer called me and invited me to join him and Kitty for a drive to Centralia, where a friend had a truck that might fit our needs. With Mitch, their wonderful chauffeur, driving, Elmer fell asleep while Kitty and I chattered away in the back seat of the Cadillac. We drove to Uhlman's Motors, a Ford and Toyota dealership in Centralia. Mr. Uhlman, clearly a good friend of Elmer's, said he had discussed our problem with Elmer, and they thought they had a solution for me. He led me over to a brand-new 1990 white Toyota four-wheel-drive truck with a canopy and a silver-blue stripe down each side. "Those are your racing stripes, Gretchen," Elmer joked as he handed me the keys. Between Mr. Uhlman and Elmer Nordstrom, the truck was a donation to Harmony Hill. I was speechless.

Driving home in this shiny, new truck that afternoon, I had to pull over to the side of the road – I couldn't see through the tears of joy that were streaming down my face. I pulled over again at Evergreen State College to show Board member Les Purce this amazing gift to Harmony Hill. His shout of joy could be heard across the campus! ❖

In the early years, Harmony Hill's Board was frequently called upon to be "hands-on." With little money and buildings of dubious stability, members of the Board often rolled up their sleeves and got a bit dirty. Mike Towey was Harmony Hill's Board president for eight years in those early days. He recruited Dick Sides to the Board and together they rounded up a group of men to undertake the restoration of the "laundry house" cabin. It was no small job. The back of the cabin had sunk eight inches into mud, the floor was collapsing, and the house was completely without insulation. Gretchen recalls that Dick brought a tractor, house-lifting jacks, railroad ties, and a few brave volunteers. They spent three full days carefully raising the building and leveling it on a foundation. Gretchen was assigned the job of keeping them well-fed and praying that the building didn't split in half when it was raised up and that the chimney didn't fall on the workers. The early Board's concerns were largely operational, and side-by-side with Gretchen they laid the groundwork for a solid future and a secure foundation. ❖

THOMAS LESLIE PURCE:
THE PEARL OF COMMUNITY

In 1989, Thomas Leslie ("Les") Purce was a new transplant to the Northwest coast, fresh from Idaho State University in Pocatello, and just settling into his position as Vice President for Advancement at Evergreen College. To get acquainted with new staff, Les sought location suggestions for a staff retreat. He was referred to a place called Harmony House.

Les has fond memories of the place: "We rented the whole upstairs of the house; Gretchen was cooking and running everything. That was the first time I talked with

Gretchen about her dreams, her plans for the future. We got to know each other, and we really hit it off. I think it was about a week or so later she called and asked if I would like to join the board.

"There was a small handful of us. I can't remember all the names now – but they were marvelous people, young and old, deeply engaged in the place. And I fell in love with Hood Canal. Well, I love oysters and crabs, too; I'd bring my boat out. The idea that you can put a pot in the water and pull up some food, it was like Christmas to me, I loved it. Still do!"

Les spent a lot of time at Harmony House. There wasn't much there yet: the lodge, the cottage, a tennis court (where the Great Hall would later be built), and the garden.

"For a while, the yurt sat on the tennis court. We had some of our early celebrations and gatherings on the court," recollects Les. "We'd set up tents and stuff. Elmer and Kitty Nordstrom would come. They were great believers in Gretchen, as were and are all of us, inspired by her vision. The Nordstroms were such marvelous, kind, generous, intelligent people. It was easy for me to get to know them because I was very close to and inspired by my grandmother, who lived to be 102. Knowing them and spending time with them – they were both in their 80s then – was like spending time with her.

"I served on one of the early boards, and as chair I negotiated the first land lease with Elmer and Kitty. We negotiated the first ten-year lease for the property, and already Gretchen was thinking about expansion," Les says with a chuckle.

"Things kind of run together in colors and fade, but I know I negotiated the second land lease when we wanted to expand and we needed public works improvements and had PERC issues and all of that stuff. We did that and then we had a grand celebration, and the Nordstroms were there. They were always so supportive. After Elmer and Kitty had both passed away, I went on to negotiate the second lease with their son John and we, too, got to be friends. John had concerns about the Hill's future, and at first, he didn't quite understand the mission as Elmer and Kitty did. Like everybody, the more he got involved, the more comfortable he became, and he brought along the next generation of Nordstrom kids.

"Then we got the Bill and Melinda Gates Foundation involved. I went to Seattle to negotiate the first half-million dollar grant for Harmony Hill with Bill Gates, Sr. Gretchen had all her work done, all laid out. She and I made a pretty good team. So we negotiated that grant, and that was really something.

"Let's see, what else? The campaign to name the bricks to get the kitchen expanded, I was involved with that. And once the kitchen was done, it wasn't big enough! Just like that," he says. He smiles broadly. "But it got people engaged. That's what it was really all about. Gretchen understood that."

Now that Les is the President of Evergreen College, he continues to bring his senior staff to Harmony Hill for annual retreats.

"Our retreats started in the yurt, then we had them in the conference space, and, after it was built, our last one was in the beautiful Great Hall. We've had many, many staff retreats on the Hill. And we have had a lot of family retreats out there, too.

"What's amazing to me is to have been in on the dream before it ever became a reality – ten years before it happened. That's how extraordinary Gretchen is. She's singularly focused and deeply humane. She doesn't use friendships, and she treats everybody the same. I just have such huge respect for her."

Les credits the early days spent at Harmony Hill and the people he met there with accelerating his acclimation to the coastal Northwest.

"I'm an interior person – high plains, desert, southern Idaho; *what Harmony Hill did for me, it really made me feel at home in Washington*. I was blessed to have some of my first best friends be some *very* extraordinary people in this state.

"I'm a lover of history and the idea of community and values, and having been friends with Kitty and Elmer was really one of the greatest blessings in my life. They'd talk about the war, when they got married, how their families first bought land, how they'd been friends since childhood when their families set up huge canvas tents to camp on the Canal before the war. Even after all their success, they were so down to earth; whenever they talked about their business, they always called it 'the shoe store.'

"We'd talk and talk, and I'd ask them all kinds of questions. All that settled me into this place, and gave me a deep, strong appreciation for what the people of the Pacific Northwest could be. Gretchen gave that to me. I loved her dream and I've always loved building, so it was fun for me to help build her dream, to be involved in the building of Harmony Hill." ❖

Long-time advisory board member **MARY WILLIAMS** recalls chairing the Harmony House personnel committee in the early years of the Hill: "Gretchen was living in the lodge, and the committee felt strongly that it was important for her to have her own living quarters. So an old, second-hand trailer was brought on the land – where the Creekside building is now – to be Gretchen's quarters. That was a *huge* step back then. I don't know if Gretchen was getting any salary or benefits at that time – very little, if any. We really made the pitch that she needed a steady salary, reasonable benefits, and more help. Gretchen did get some part-time kitchen help, and maybe had a gardening helper once in a while, but there was no full-time staff there in those days.

"I've enjoyed just watching it grow," Mary continues. "It's so different now, with the new buildings, but it's also very much the same; it has the same feel. When I first saw the drawings, I thought, 'Oh, it's going to be ruined, it'll never be the same.' But it still has the same aura about it for me. It still feels like home.

"In the early days, Gretchen would share her vision and most of us couldn't see it yet. We'd say, 'Yeah, okay, Gretchen, that's nice.' She was undeterred, though. She has such strength and conviction. Just step aside, and don't get in her way. I still just shake my head. I can't believe this all happened. I never should have doubted it would." ❖

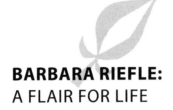

BARBARA RIEFLE:
A FLAIR FOR LIFE

"I would like to believe when I die that I have given myself away like a tree that sows seeds every spring and never counts the loss, because it is not loss, it is adding to future life. It is the tree's way of being. Strongly rooted, perhaps, but spilling out its treasure on the wind."

– QUOTE FROM A MAY SARTON ESSAY,
READ AT BARBARA RIEFLE'S MEMORIAL SERVICE

In the center of the circular drive that carries visitors to and from Harmony Hill's Lodge stands a small flowering cherry tree, its multitude of long, graceful branches extending in all directions. It was planted by a group of remarkable friends to honor an exceptional woman, Barbara Riefle. The group calls itself the FOBs (Friends of Barbara), and the tree reminds them of her generous spirit, how she reached out and connected to so many. And Barbara continues to touch the lives of every person who is able to attend a cancer retreat at no cost because of her dream to give everyone that choice.

Barbara loved having choices. She made a number of good choices from the time she was on her own at age eighteen and both her parents were deceased. She held a full time job as she worked her way through college, eventually earning a Master's degree at Columbia University. She married Hank Riefle and bought a small travel agency in her beloved New York City. The Riefles developed the tiny four-person firm into a highly-successful company with over two hundred employees. Respected and admired as a smart, innovative businesswoman, Barbara was beloved for personal qualities: she was passionate about her city, about travel, food and wine, the arts, and most of all, about her abundant family of friends.

Friend Helena Cohen recalls, "Every one of us thought we were her best friend. That's how she made you feel."

Helena met Barbara in 1986, when she had moved from South Africa to New York City. They clicked right away – sharing many tastes, interests, and a love of travel. They remained lifelong friends, even after Helena moved to the West Coast.

"In 2000, I got a call from Barbara about her diagnosis of appendix cancer. She came out and stayed with me; it was shortly after she'd had surgery, and her prognosis was poor – she was given three to six months to live. Her life turned on a dime. We drove out to Harmony Hill, 'out in the boonies.' I remember sitting with her on the swing in this peaceful, embracing place. I took her to her room. Having traveled with Barbara to some pretty high-end places, I didn't know how she'd like the rather spare lodging. She noted they didn't even have matching towels," Helena says, smiling at the recollection. "I told her if she wanted to leave, she could just call and I would come get her. Having the choice helped her stay – she didn't *have* to. And after that three-day retreat, she was absolutely *transformed*."

Barbara was living with cancer by the time Marjorie Luckey met her.

"She felt that Harmony Hill had really given her life back. Barbara was the most alive person that I have ever met, with or without cancer," says Marjorie. "She was so joyous about life – totally engaged with people, with events, with culture, with friends, in the leadership development conference; it was quite a remarkable phenomenon to know her. Here was someone who was dying and, while she would occasionally talk about death, she was living every day, intensely and joyously. She attributed that to her experience at Harmony Hill, and she was a major supporter of the Hill. It was in tribute to Barbara that I later decided to participate as a housemother there."

Elaine Holland and Barbara met through mutual friends and a *Future Thinking* development conference.

Elaine shares her memories of Barbara: "She was a very, *very* special person. After she got sick, she became obsessed with eating right, putting the right things into her body. She came into all the FOBs kitchens and threw out everything that was unhealthy, got us into rice cakes and tahini and all the fresh vegetables and the right way to cook. That was just another of her gifts to us – a refinement for some of us, and for some, a whole new way of cooking and eating."

"She was appalled by the lack of information about cancer, about the lack of choices," says Helena. "She went all out, really put her organizational skills to work, to find out everything she could about appendix cancer. She became a spokesperson. Harmony Hill was such a great resource for her; she could accept her diagnosis and share the resources."

Marjorie, a physician, recollects, "When I first met Barbara, I thought I was going to be able to help her in some way because I was a physician, and I really understood the medical system. Turned out about six months after we became friends, I was diagnosed with colon cancer, and it was *she* who helped *me*.

"She was the one I would call when I was just feeling rotten and angry and in moods I didn't want other people to see; times when I felt weak, angry, vulnerable and also guilty because I felt all of those things. Guilty, too, because I knew that my cancer was curable and hers was not. She was an amazing friend during that period: always listening with compassion to whatever I was feeling; providing information about cancer resources like massage, restorative yoga, acupuncture and meditation; and helping me come to terms with my diagnosis. She was a rock and an inspiration during that time."

Elaine remembers going to a New Year's Eve party at Barbara's, where "we were all talking about the impact Harmony Hill had on her attitude after her cancer diagnosis. We were all feeling enthused, and when I offered to run a marathon to raise funds for a big, well-known cancer hospital, Barbara blurted out, 'Why run for a big place while Harmony Hill doesn't even have matching towels!'"

Elaine and Barbara called Gretchen about their plan, and Elaine ran the next New York Marathon to raise funds for Harmony Hill.

"We thought we'd raise $5,000 but we raised $10,000! The second year, we raised $23,000; the third year, $35,000. And that was the year Barbara suggested I join the Harmony Hill Board. As a result of the NYC Marathon fundraising plan, Harmony Hill was able to start offering the cancer retreats at no charge, a landmark moment in its history.

"That summer in 2002, when we raised the $35,000, Barbara was very ill. Her nurse pulled me aside and said, 'You keep talking about that marathon in the fall… she may not make it.' But it gave Barbara something to focus on, rather than cancer, cancer, cancer. She loved it. We had a whole program where we'd sign people up, send personal letters. I'd say to Barbara, 'I know you're sick, but these letters are a royal pain. If you could just hang in there for one more marathon….' It became a joke between us."

"Barbara managed her cancer by saying, 'I live with cancer,' not 'I have cancer,' says Helena. "It was important to her to be able to choose how and on what she spent her precious time. And she was so thoughtful, always sending a handwritten note or a small gift of remembrance; she always showed so much class in everything she did."

"Towards the end of her life, she wasn't able to go out and shop or have dinner, any of those things she used to do," Elaine says. "And one of her doctors told her that you 'learn to appreciate what you can appreciate now.' Barbara called me one day and said, 'Oh it's a horrible day; it's raining.' And then she caught herself and said, 'Wait, no, it's a wonderful day. And it happens to be raining.'

"Now that's one thing that we FOBs do, we catch ourselves and say, 'No, it's a wonderful day. And it happens to be snowing.'"

The day after the 2002 New York Marathon, Barbara slipped into a coma and died soon after.

"After she passed away, I got a box," says Helena. "A lot of people got little boxes; she had sent us each gifts. She knew I loved roses, and she gave me a crystal rose vase that she had gotten for her wedding. She was incredibly generous."

Marjorie talks about how important the FOBs are to one another: "Most of us had met but we weren't tightly connected until Barbara's death. We sat around at her home after she had died, and we realized that there were these wonderful people that we had gotten to know through taking care of her the last few months; and we didn't want to lose touch."

"After Barbara's death, we started meeting once a month in New York City for

"Love doesn't mean doing extraordinary or heroic things. It means knowing how to do ordinary things with tenderness."

– JEAN VANIER

lunch," says Elaine. "And we have met for a four- or five-hour lunch every month since she died in 2002. So the gift Barbara had of touching everyone's lives is sustained. The FOBs have been supportive of the Hill over the years – fundraising and volunteering in various ways. We consider ourselves very fortunate to have this relationship with each other and with Harmony Hill.

"I'm glad for the FOBs, that I still have that connection with them and with Barbara," Helena says. *"She would be so proud of Harmony Hill's continuation. Service was her gift. And she lives on."* ❖

ELAINE HOLLAND:
RUNNING FOR A REASON

Elaine Holland, one of the FOBs, is a mover and shaker. A highly-successful businesswoman, global citizen and worldwide marathon runner, she's served on the Harmony Hill Board of Directors for eight years and will lead the Board as President in 2012.

Born and raised in Oregon, Elaine moved with her family every two years because her dad worked for the state. She attended Goucher College on a scholarship in Baltimore. An art major with a chemistry minor, she restored paintings for two months after graduation and discovered she hated it. When she took a job waitressing and found she loved it, she thought, "Oh, my dear, I've gone astray!

"I moved back to Portland, took a sales job and was lucky enough to get on with IBM," Elaine recalls. "And I worked for them for 16 years."

With IBM, Elaine moved from Portland to Denver, then to Albuquerque, and after that, to Atlanta. She then recruited to British Telecom, eventually was promoted and moved to London to become the general manager of their computing electronics sectors, with offices in Munich, Paris and London. After three years, she moved back to New York and joined Perot Systems. There she became reacquainted with Barbara Riefle, with whom she developed an abiding friendship.

After 28 years in technology, Elaine was ready for something different. She became an executive recruiter for Heidrick and Struggles; from there, she joined WPP, a world leader in marketing communications. After two years at the Group level, Elaine joined one of WPP's operating companies, Millward Brown, a global marketing research agency, where she led global talent for six years. Recently, she became the Senior Vice President of Executive Coaching & Development, supporting the development of the senior executive team.

Elaine's passions, however, are not limited to the world of high-powered business. She's also competitive in the realm of personal bests, completing 17 marathons in various cities in the U.S. Recently, she has set a goal to join the "50-States Marathon Club" by completing marathons in all fifty states.

In 2000, when she and Barbara Riefle hatched their plan for Harmony Hill fundraising via marathon runs, Elaine was looking forward to reaping more than endorphins at the end of that year's New York City Marathon. The first year's marathon raised more than double their goal; the next year four times that. In 2002, Elaine, joined by her 77-year-old athletic mother, Maree Rushlow (herself a cancer survivor), ran the New York Marathon, and $35,000 was raised that year. After Barbara's death, the annual Harmony Hill marathon fundraiser was named in her honor: The Barbara Riefle Scholarship Fund. Elaine has continued to run every fall for the fund, and marathon donors have contributed over $100,000 so far – providing the opportunity for people living with cancer to experience the valuable support that Barbara found at a Harmony Hill cancer retreat.

In addition to Elaine's marathons, five other New York City FOBs, Barbara Gallay, Tricia Newell, Kate Duncan, Janet Peek, and Hank Riefle, continue to support and raise funds for Harmony Hill.

Elaine, along with her cats Fred, Gloria and Chet, recently moved back to Portland to be near her 84-year-old mother. She's also looking forward to being on the grounds of Harmony Hill more often than she was while living in New York.

"Harmony Hill has always been 'hallowed ground' to me. Barbara used to say 'If God had a living room, this would be it.' During my very first visit to the Hill, a celebration was taking place; a group of cancer-retreat graduates was meeting to share stories about their experiences. One of them, Julie Ziegler, an artist and a lovely young lady, made gorgeous hanging murals from all kinds of paper, graphics, and calligraphy as thank-you gifts for the Harmony Hill Board. After she was diagnosed, she had lost her ability to create. She reclaimed it after being at Harmony Hill. Julie's artistic creations are so beautiful; I was touched deeply by her artistry and her generosity.

"As I sat there listening to the participants talking about their lives, it struck me that *the gift of cancer is the awareness of the importance of every day. And there's no reason we have to get cancer to learn that lesson*. We can learn that lesson without having the experience of cancer. I frequently reflect on what another alumnus, Marge Putman, shared about creating her own space for herself – a place for her books, her reading area, her place of meditation – and again, I was so moved by the fact that she'd reclaimed her own life for herself as part of her healing. She inspired me to reflect on my life and to realize that I wasn't taking care of myself as well as I should.

"Marge also walked the New York City Marathon to raise money for the scholarship fund. And Karen Schrantz of Seattle, who attends yoga retreats at Harmony Hill, ran the Seattle Marathon to fundraise for the Hill, too. So this whole idea of doing a marathon to raise much-needed funds has expanded and flourished beyond my actions and Barbara's dreams." ❖

"Wherever there is a human being, there is an opportunity for kindness."

– SENECA

By the new millennium, the Harmony Hill Board's focus had shifted from operational to strategic. With an ever-growing and capable staff, there was far less need for the Board to take on physical responsibilities. More than ever, the Board focused its attention on the important task of raising funds to support the mission. Where once a grant of $50,000 was manna from heaven, the size of the financial goals grew as Harmony Hill's vision grew. Susan Keith, Board president in 2002-2003, became the chair of the Major Gift Taskforce in 2006. Its goal was to raise $1.5 million by then end of 2008. If that goal was met, matching funds of $500,000 would be granted by the Bill & Melinda Gates Foundation. As the deadline approached – with only six months to go – Harmony Hill was still $750,000 short of its goal and the economy had entered a downturn. Leaders met with fundraising guru Lynne Twist, author of *The Soul of Money.* She offered inspiration and coaching which injected new ideas and renewed energy into the Taskforce. It came down to the wire, but on December 31, 2008, Harmony Hill's Board, volunteers, and staff celebrated the successful realization of their goal.

Today, in addition to the ever-present quest for funding, Harmony Hill's Board takes seriously its responsibility to create a sustainable and expansive vision for the Hill. Beyond the current cancer retreats, which will always be at the center of Harmony Hill's mission, the Board has a vision of expanded programs for children, health care professionals, and taking an active, leadership role in a new initiative for global health. ❖

CAROLYN OLSEN:
FOREVER AMAZED

Carolyn Olsen and Gretchen Schodde met on a hay bale in Eastern Washington. "I was on the Mason-Thurston County's Drug and Alcohol Abuse Prevention Board, and we were both in Eastern Washington at a conference on drug and alcohol abuse. We struck up a conversation and found out that we're from the same town."

They planned to get together when they got back home from the conference. Carolyn lives in Shelton, and Gretchen was then staying at St. Andrew's.

"I went out to St. Andrew's and Gretchen told me she knew she had this calling – she wanted to have a retreat center, and the house next door to St. Andrew's was available. And I said, 'Dream on, Sweetheart.' It wasn't but a short time later that she was renting the laundry room over there. I thought, 'This woman is unbelievable.' And then she got into the big house! She's one of those people who just draw you in, and I started being filled up with the hope that she had that she could actually achieve this tremendous idea. And so I've kind of been there with her for twenty years.

"I've been on the Board a couple of times; I'm still on the advisory board. Sometimes a couple months may go by since the last Hill project I was involved with, and then Gretchen will call and say, 'Can you help me with this?' And I'll drive back out there and get out of my car, look around, and say, 'Oh my God, why haven't I been back out here for so long!' It just does that *thing* to your heart and your body, just the beauty of the place.

"Most projects that happen out there are definitely dear to my heart and I want to see them succeed, so I try to participate and help as much as I can.

"Gretchen just has that effect on people; you just feel like you want to make things easier so she can get on with this business. Because everybody knows that whatever is happening out at the Hill is important.

"I've been doing things at the Hill forever. And my husband Rod was a silent participant. Whatever I wanted to do out there was fine, and he would wave me on....

"When he had mylodysplastic anemia, and was getting chemo and going through all this stuff, Gretchen would beg for him to please come out for a cancer retreat. And I would say, 'Gretchen, you know he's not going to want to do that, but I'll keep asking.' So I kept asking, and one day he said yes. I said, 'You only have to stay half a day, it'll be a quick in-and-outer, and maybe you'll learn something.' So we went out there and we sat in a circle of people who were living with cancer and their caregivers, and all of a sudden my husband just started to spill his feelings and what was happening to him. Because he felt comfortable and safe enough to be able to share what was going on. And I learned things about his journey that I'd had no clue, absolutely no clue, whatsoever about. He stayed for lunch, and he continued talking. Though he couldn't make himself stay the rest of the day, the fact that he went and that he actually shared his journey was miraculous. I will forever be open-mouthed and amazed that this happened for him.

"So things that happen on the Hill are unbelievable, unbelievable. I've seen people walk in the door dying – literally dying – as they walk in the door, and three short days later, walk out with hope in their eyes and making plans for a reunion with the people that they've met. And they're dying. It's just amazing.

"*There isn't a person who goes to the Hill, no matter who they are, that doesn't leave with something that's a positive in their lives.* Not a person. And I don't care if they're just delivering milk."

Long before she became the owner of Sage Bookstore in Shelton, Carolyn went to school to become a nurse, but ended up being a surgical tech and working for a doctor.

"I always worked in something to do with medicine. Then I was a homemaker, raised five beautiful babies, and accidentally became a bookstore owner. I was president of the chamber of commerce when I came into this building to talk to the landowner. I said, 'You have this empty space; we want to help you build.' And he said,

'Well, we need a bookstore,' and I said, 'Oh, my God, yes we do'! Then he said, 'Why don't *you* put one in here?'

"I was a very unsophisticated mystery-book reader, so my first thought was how could I possibly?" Carolyn laughs her big, easy laugh, "Well, I've now been here seven years. We have too big an inventory, and it doesn't make any money, but I just love books so much. I keep buying them and putting them up here. We have 20,000 books; for a town this size, that's pretty good."

Carolyn's bookstore provides the books that Harmony Hill sells in its gift shop.

"I try to give big enough discount so they can sell and make some money. And we sell Harmony Hill's cookbook here. We also participate when Ann Lovejoy is conducting workshops at the Hill – we sell books for her, and we give Harmony Hill a 20 percent donation, so it works out."

Besides working together for Harmony Hill, Carolyn and Gretchen have done some terrific traveling together.

"I was able to go to China with her as part of a People-to-People tour, and I went to Iona, Scotland, with her," says Carolyn. "She's become part of my life; she's just like a sister."

When asked what's special about Gretchen, Carolyn replies without hesitation, "She has a naïve simplicity about her – but she's also so worldly. We've also joked about her being the Mother Teresa of Mason County. She's just so unassuming and so grateful. And she's one of the funniest women, ever. She isn't all seriousness, she's really funny. But you don't ever want to get stuck with her and her purse. Getting her through customs in China was …." Carolyn rolls her eyes. "She has *everything* in her purse: throat lozenges, Ayurvedic stuff, arnica, papers from the last Harmony Hill event. She's a paper-and-stuff collector. Everything is important to her. Everything." ❖

> "Love the moment. Flowers grow out of dark moments. Therefore, each moment is vital. It affects the whole. Life is a succession of such moments and to live each, is to succeed."
>
> – CORITA KENT

Friends come on four feet as well as on two. Among the many creatures that live at or frequent the Hill, Cali is certainly the most beloved. A calico cat who has been "queen of the hill" since 1999, she is an integral part of the hospitality team. She loves to walk the labyrinth with guests, or accompany them on hikes. Herself a cancer survivor, Cali seems to know who among a group most needs her company. She will happily curl at their feet or in their laps, her soft purring harmonizing with the conversation around her.

Gretchen recalls the first time she saw Cali – a tiny kitten sprinting across the porch of the Lodge. "We did what you always do with a small animal, we fed her. And, of course, she's been here ever since.

"When she'd been with us for about a year, Cali developed an acute respiratory ailment that was very frightening. I rushed her to the vet who diagnosed her with cancer of the lungs. He sent us home with prednisone, which he said would help with her symptoms, but warned that she would probably only last a couple of months. When I told our staff of Cali's prognosis, they were terribly upset, many in tears. Someone suggested that we establish a support group for her, like the ones that have been formed for so many of our cancer retreat participants."

They did exactly that. They put the word out into the community to send Cali healing thoughts. Over the next few months, there were periodic "Cali congregations," and she was included in many prayer circles both near and far. In only a few weeks, it appeared to the folks at Harmony Hill that Cali was getting stronger each day, not weaker as the veterinarian had forecast. Gretchen took her back to the vet who couldn't believe how well she was doing. That was more than ten years ago. And while Cali has had countless scrapes and close-calls over the years, she continues to thrive in the healing atmosphere of Harmony Hill.

One day, many years ago, Gretchen was deeply touched to watch Cali follow a cancer retreat participant as she slowly walked the labyrinth.

"When she came to the center, she sat weeping for quite some time. I watched from my office window. Cali sat by the woman's side the entire time and she kept rubbing her own eyes with her paws – it looked as though Cali was weeping, too. Such a precious sharing I was witnessing!"

Cali has also perfected the art of becoming the center of attention at events large and small. Hill staffer Cindy Shank was married at Harmony Hill some years ago. As the wedding procession walked across the lawn, Cali leaped in front of Cindy in mad pursuit of a mouse...which she, of course, caught. Some guests speculated that it was Cali's way of stealing the show, others contended that she merely wanted everything to be perfect for Cindy's day. After all, in a cat's world, the presence of a mouse simply cannot be tolerated. ❖

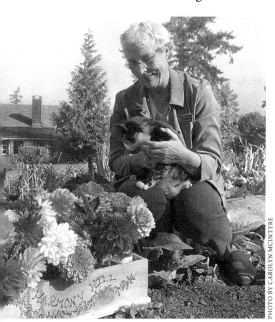

Gretchen and Cali the cat.

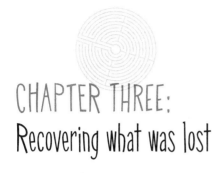

CHAPTER THREE:
Recovering what was lost

"By the time I got to Harmony Hill, my sense of myself as a person had been erased by procedure after procedure of cancer treatments. My sense of dignity was totally gone. I was really struggling with my sense of self. I needed to re-member myself, put myself back together. (During the program) I started feeling like a person again for the first time in a very long time. There was no pity – that doesn't help move us forward – but a genuine compassion. The whole experience was totally life changing. The experience of the retreat and the healing that happened went so deep that I carry it with me now throughout my life. It has sustained me through some very hard times since then. I thought cancer was the beginning of the end for me. I discovered, through the retreat, that this wasn't so. The retreat gave me back my life. I was willing to begin again."

– JULIE BARRETT ZIEGLER, 2000 HARMONY HILL ALUMNA

In 1990, Harmony House changed its name to Harmony Hill. As the buildings expanded and the mission became clearer, the new name better reflected its evolution. Harmony Hill was a place where people could reconnect with themselves and with the earth. It was a place of conscious living, healing and spiritual renewal. It was more than a house – it was a community inspired by love and wholeness. ❧

JULIE BARRETT ZIEGLER:
LOSING WHAT MATTERS MOST

"My first language isn't English, it's color, and that was lost to me during my treatment for cancer." For Julie Barrett Ziegler, a prolific artist and teacher, art was her oxygen and sustenance before cancer. She was diagnosed with breast cancer in 1999. After surgery, chemo, and radiation, Julie fell into a deep and cavernous depression.

She completely lost touch with her art and the fulfillment she had always received from it. She describes that time as "ugly, dark, terrifying and horrible – I was suicidal, ready to check out."

Julie's experience of the medical system was dehumanizing. "I was a diagnosis, a procedure, a patient number. I wasn't a name or an individual. I saw dozens of medical professionals. Almost nobody looked me in the eye and saw me for who I was, except for one amazing doctor and my awesome chemo nurse, who actually spent time with me. I see now that many of the medical professionals were as burned out as I was by the system they worked in, but by the end of all the treatment and drugs I felt devalued to the point where I didn't care if I lived or died. My family was in turmoil, my art was gone, I'd lost my job and my income."

For Julie, treatment for cancer was worse than the actual disease. She decided to discontinue treatment, regardless of what the ultimate outcome might be. Her doctor was at a loss for how to treat the bottomless depression Julie was experiencing. She recommended Harmony Hill.

"My first thought upon arriving there was, 'This is a place of intention.' From the moment I entered, I felt received, I felt genuinely welcomed.

"We were all tended to on so many levels. It wasn't just one thing that broke through to me, it was the atmosphere that said *you're in charge of your healing – we're just here to help.*"

Julie notes that it was profound to be asked "What do you want?" – so unlike her experience of the medical system proceeding in heedless disregard of the patient's wishes or concerns.

"After three days at Harmony Hill, I felt whole again. To be held with such caring and intention was what did it. I felt I'd been given back my name, I'd found my soul again.

"I was a different person when I came back home. My family recognized it immediately. We cried together over dinner that night. It was such a powerful and healing experience for all of us."

With overpowering gratitude, Julie started making blessing banners for Gretchen, Melissa, and the other program leaders at Harmony Hill. "I made six or seven in the space of two weeks and knew then that my inner eye was open again. Inspiration was everywhere. My art – the thing that moves my heart and makes me tick – was restored to me. I found my passion and purpose again. I found my self…and I started healing."

In the intervening years, Julie has returned to Harmony Hill occasionally as a teacher and facilitator, leading groups in the creation of prayer banners and art therapy. She has also become a hospice volunteer, playing her harp for people who are dying and their families.

"I stopped thinking about dying and became focused on living. That was the gift each of us received at Harmony Hill. Whether we had three months to live, three years, or thirty, when we left, each of us knew *how we were going to live.* How many other people have been given that gift?"

Today, Julie's studio is a banquet of colors, textures, and evocative images, ranging from the sacred to the whimsical. Julie's art reflects her healing and her gratitude. It shines with the same inner light that she has. Her gift is also Harmony Hill's gift: the ability to be awake and aware and focused on living.

"Harmony Hill helped me see my cancer not as a burden but as an initiation to a deeper and more purposeful life.

"Harmony Hill gave me permission to be the author of my own life. Don't let anyone tell you that because you have cancer your life is being ripped away. Pursue whatever lifts your heart." ❖

GRETCHEN:
OPENING TO MIRACLES

My mom has been a three-time cancer survivor (breast cancer in 1966 and again in 1999). In 1990, a routine dental check-up detected a tumor that was later diagnosed as malignant by an oral surgeon. We consulted with numerous doctors, a couple of whom wanted to hospitalize her immediately and perform radical neck surgery. Fortunately, we found Dr. Glenn Warner, who was Kitty Nordstrom's oncologist. He was viewed as unconventional and there was controversy around him, but he was just what we needed at the time. He encouraged us as a family to get a grip on our stress. He said the cancer didn't come overnight and we didn't need to take care of it overnight. So my folks went fishing; my brother and sister sought calming activities, and I did what relaxes me most: I headed to the garden.

It was spring, and time to rototill. The hardest thing about rototilling is just getting the heavy, awkward machine started. Once I did that, however, I found I was having difficulty tilling in straight lines as I had always done before. A question suddenly came to me: *Why must I till in straight lines?* Internally, I granted the rototiller permission to go in any way it wanted and said that I would follow. I stopped hanging on so tightly and found that I was tilling in wide circles. Very soon I realized I was making a circle garden – which years later became the labyrinth garden. As I approached center, I had the realization that letting go of control and trusting the direction I was taking could be applied to so much more than this garden task.

When our family regrouped to address Mom's cancer, we agreed upon a surgical procedure somewhat less radical than the doctors had suggested earlier. Nonetheless, it was a major surgery. I accompanied Mom to see the head and neck surgeon on the top floor of the Nordstrom Tower at Swedish. The surgeon examined my mother closely, he looked at me, and then back at her. "You are weird," he said to us both.

"I beg your pardon?" What a peculiar thing for a surgeon to say to us!

"You're weird," he repeated. "Take a look." I had seen the grayish black tumor at the back of Mom's molars, but when I looked this time, all I saw was pink, healthy tissue. The tumor was completely gone. The surgeon couldn't believe it. He couldn't get us out of there fast enough because he didn't know how to deal with this development. If only he had felt comfortable enough to explore this example of spontaneous healing. If only he had asked, "What did you do? Tell me everything." Sadly, it was beyond the scope of his comprehension or his view of reality to do that.

We were ecstatic! Practically dancing with joy as we went down the elevator. We called my dad from the lobby; he was thrilled beyond words. We also called Kitty Nordstrom and she invited us to come right over and celebrate.

I tell this story often at cancer retreats. Miracles do happen. We hear about such things but never think they could happen to us. But they do. My mother experienced what was truly a spontaneous and complete remission. It opened my mind to all the possibilities out there, and I hope her story can do the same for others. ❖

> "There are only two ways to live your life.
> One is as though nothing is a miracle The other
> is as though everything is a miracle."
>
> – ALBERT EINSTEIN

GRETCHEN:
A NEW BEGINNING FOR HARMONY HILL

The Commonweal Cancer Program was featured on the last part of the Bill Moyers PBS special about "Healing and the Mind." I was spellbound when I watched it, having just been through my mom's cancer experience. If we had known about Commonweal, we would surely have tried to go there.

After I saw the PBS special, I couldn't quit thinking about Commonweal. Finally, a few weeks later I called them. They had been inundated with calls – hundreds from all across the country. A wise decision had been made when they started their program, to offer it no more than six times a year – they knew how intense it was, and how easily facilitators could experience burnout. They wanted always to be able to look forward to the next session. Also, they limited their program to eight attendees. It was clear that learning about Commonweal had touched a chord for so many people and that they were being called (quite literally!) to another level of service. They launched what they termed "Tradecraft" – a workshop designed to share what they had learned with other centers which were interested in replicating it. They did not want to create a franchise, but shared whatever they could to help other centers. As you might imagine, there was a lot of competition to get into this program. Harmony Hill was fortunate to be accepted into the very first training and went on to become one of the five most active programs in the country inspired by the Commonweal model.

I was blessed to be part of that first training and mentored by co-founder Rachel Remen, MD. I also met with Dr. Michael Lerner, her partner in creating Commonweal. These are two of the most remarkable people I have ever known. Each time I revisit Commonweal, I marvel at their astounding spirits, their profound commitment to healing, and the wonderful staff they recruit. I am filled with gratitude for the many angels along the path that led to this new beginning for Harmony Hill. ❖

Participants in Harmony Hill's Cancer Program find strength, resiliency, camaraderie, and healing in the retreats. While cure may not be an outcome for some participants, healing happens in many different ways. Through group sharing and support sessions, creative arts, gentle movement, and exploration of lifestyle choices and strategies, attendees gain new perspective on their illness and tools to help them move forward to manage their health. Equally important, the retreats provide a setting to explore feelings and questions that people with cancer often have but haven't been able to voice in a safe and nurturing environment.

In 2004, the Harmony Hill Board of Directors made the decision to offer the cancer and caregiver retreats free of charge to attendees. They recognized that even a modest registration fee was a barrier for many people who were facing the challenge of a cancer diagnosis, or of caring for a loved one with cancer. Even with good insurance, out-of-pocket costs and lost wages create a financial burden for many, and the notion of spending money to attend a cancer retreat is improbable. The Board did not want anyone to be excluded from Harmony Hill due to financial constraints, nor did they want money worries to overshadow the benefits of the experience. ❖

PATRICK AND SARAH HEALY:
NO MORE MASQUERADE

Sometimes it takes a while for healing to happen.

Patrick Healy was diagnosed with non-Hodgkin's lymphoma in 2002. During 2002 and 2003, he endured arduous treatment and he faced it pretty much alone. Friends disappeared in the face of their own fears or not knowing the "right" thing to say. Because he was a big, strong guy, Patrick's doctor told him that in addition to surgery, he would be getting "maximum strength" chemo and radiation. Even so, the doctor said, Patrick's chances of living beyond 2004 were slight.

That's a lot to face for anyone, even a guy who rides motorcycles and looks pretty tough to the outside world. And so he went to chemo alone and he came home alone to an empty house. He kept everything inside – the fears, the loneliness, the anger – and he waited for 2004, he waited for his own death.

The year 2004 came and Patrick didn't die. In fact, his body was recovering from the onslaught of the cancer and the treatment for it.

"In a way, I was disappointed that I didn't die. I really didn't have any reason to live. I had lost my job and nobody was going to hire a guy with cancer. I had lost any perspective on life. It was all about death."

If death wasn't going to come for him, Patrick started seeking it out: "I started doing some pretty reckless things. Riding my Harley way too fast and hanging out with the wrong kind of people."

Finally, one friend helped him face his self-destructive behavior.

"He told me, 'You're killing yourself, and I don't want you to die.' I needed to hear that. It meant so much to me. *Somebody cared*."

Patrick turned his energy to the motorcycle club he had founded in 2002, "Bikers Fighting Cancer." During his treatment he had met an 11-year-old boy, Ray, who was fighting brain cancer. His biggest wish was to be in a motorcycle club, so together they started up Bikers Fighting Cancer. Ray designed a logo and coined the motto "Never Give Up." Ray died in 2004 and was buried in his leather vest with the club patch. Patrick redoubled his efforts to build the club. BFC held rallies and sold t-shirts and other merchandise, with all of the money raised going to help children and families struggling in the face of cancer.

Today there are hundreds of members in Bikers Fighting Cancer motorcycle clubs in several chapters throughout the western states. It was at a club event in Bellingham, Washington, where Patrick met Sarah in 2007. She bought a t-shirt from him and they talked about the BFC mission of helping kids with cancer.

"I could see he was special, and also that he was very sad," she recalls.

"When I met her," Patrick says, "I was dead inside. She gave me a reason to live, and the healing started." Patrick shared some of his poetry with Sarah. He let her see his fears and his vulnerability, and she remained by his side, encouraging him to reveal his emotions, no matter what they were. Sarah and Patrick were married in 2009.

Late in 2009, Sarah happened to see an article about Harmony Hill in *The Seattle Times*. While reading it, she recalls, "I knew in my heart that this was what Patrick needed. I hoped it would help him to work through all those years of treatment and of being alone; I hoped it would lessen the pain that he still carried, the sadness. I didn't realize that Harmony Hill was for me, too, until we got there. It was what we *both* needed."

"I was scared to go," Patrick admits. "There was stuff inside that I had never let out. I didn't know if I could let it out, or if I wanted to. Even filling out the application was hard – putting into words what I had been through. I was crying the whole time. But Sarah's given me the confidence that it's okay to cry and it's okay to feel. We went, but I was afraid. "

During the first afternoon of the retreat, participants share in circle what they have been going through in their journey with cancer or as a caregiver. Patrick volunteered to go first, certain he was the most afraid of anyone in the room. Telling his story of treatment, and of loneliness and fear, the tears flowed freely. For Patrick, opening the circle at Harmony Hill turned out to be his own opening, as well.

"I let out emotions I had been holding tight inside for so long. I said what I was feeling and nobody judged me. I was accepted for who I was. I cried a lot during those three days, and it was okay.

"A lot of men have been raised by fathers like my own, fathers who taught their sons it's not okay to cry. It's not manly. That's a hard lesson to unlearn, but it's freeing.

"At one point in the retreat I was able to voice my greatest fear of all, that Sarah might leave me – tired at last of dealing with my fears and my cancer. Others shared that they had the same fear of losing the person they loved most. This is all so hard on the caregiver."

Sarah's eyes shine with love as she looks at him and says softly, "I'm not going anywhere."

She continues, "I went to Harmony Hill for him, but I came away with so much for myself. I saw that I wasn't alone in what I was feeling. Other caregivers were facing the same fears and uncertainty. I felt so much support from other participants, and from the Harmony Hill staff."

"Harmony Hill is a place of total acceptance," says Patrick. "It was okay to do whatever we felt like doing, and to say whatever we were feeling. We made jokes that wouldn't be acceptable – or understood – elsewhere. It was also a very spiritual experience, though not, for me, in a religious sense. Each of us touched our spirit in our own way. It showed me how to go deeper, to reach far into my soul.

"I've carried that with me since Harmony Hill. I haven't closed the door that opened there. I'm willing to show my emotions, to be honest and to be vulnerable. Cancer turned my world upside-down, at first in a very bad way. Now, though, I see all

> **"**In the depth of winter I finally learned that within me there lay an invincible summer."
>
> – ALBERT CAMUS

the good things it's brought. Sarah is number one, plus we have great new friends and a far less materialistic lifestyle. We have a rich life.

"Before cancer, I was living a lie – thinking that a big house and a new car were the most important things in the world. They meant that I was successful, I could provide for my family. But cancer taught me that's not what life's about. Cancer introduced me to friends who had next to nothing, but they were happy to share what little they had. They knew how to be happy."

Today Patrick and Sarah have downsized their home and moved to the Olympic Peninsula. They're only a few mlles from Harmony Hill and are already working with Gretchen on creating a new retreat for children who have a parent or sibling with cancer.

"These kids can be forgotten, with so much attention on their family member with cancer. It's hard for them. We want to create a place where they feel safe to talk about whatever they're feeling and where they can be with other kids who share their experiences."

It's been a long ride for Patrick since his diagnosis in 2002. But it's brought him to just where he wants to be: "I've learned what matters. I've learned to be happy." ❖

Every cancer retreat at Harmony Hill is different from every other. Each one evolves in response to the people who are there – their needs, their concerns, their interactions. One thing that doesn't change is the circle that opens each retreat. Each participant is invited to tell his or her cancer story, from diagnosis – or even before – to arrival at Harmony Hill. The story can be as long or as short as the teller wants. They hold a token, or "talking stick" – often it's a large heart-shaped rock that was given to Gretchen some years ago. There are no interruptions, no judgments. For some, it's the first time they have been able to tell their story, or to voice certain fears, or perhaps been listened to with attention and acceptance. Whether speaking or listening, there are often tears, and just as often laughter.

There is a kind of magic in the circle that opens each retreat at Harmony Hill. Not the sleight-of-hand magic we see on stages, but the quiet, everyday magic that reminds us how connected we are, and opens up doors and windows that we had lost awareness of. ❖

GRETCHEN:
THE OPENING CIRCLE

The opening circle of our cancer retreats always reminds me of a mosaic. It's like a grand and powerful mystery: every person shows up how and when they should. And as they connect, something beautiful is made whole. The mosaic comes together as something breathtakingly beautiful. Each person is here because they are meant to be here. And we all seem to know that we have so much to learn from one another. What each has to share is as important as anything we offer in our program curriculum – perhaps even more so.

I always feel honored to welcome our participants in the opening circle. There is an amazing bonding that begins – a recognition and kinship among these fellow travelers. Often participants come with fears, anger, confusion, and hope – all of which is held safely in the circle.

One of the quotes I use a lot is an anonymous one – I wish I knew the source: "Life is not about waiting for the storms to pass, it is about learning to dance in the rain." (We actually have this on the back of one of our t-shirts now since it is used so frequently and resonates so deeply.)

I also usually tell about a research project that was done with some hikers who were given a weight to put in their backpack before climbing a steep hill. At the top they were asked how heavy they thought the weight was and how steep the hill was. Consistently, those who walked with a friend believed the load was lighter and the hill was less steep. This, I tell the cancer retreat participants, is our hope for the weekend: when they leave here the load will feel lighter and the path less steep, and they'll have some new tools for the journey.

When we first started these programs I was concerned about needing to match participants by something: diagnosis, prognosis, age, etc. I was worried that someone who had just been diagnosed would be upset to be around someone who was clearly nearing the end of their days. I called Waz Thomas, Commonweal's program manager, and asked his advice. He told me, "Don't try to match people…trust that the right ones will show up at the right time." This brilliant advice has guided us as we have served more than 120 extended care retreats. Every time, I witness how the light in their lives that may have been dimmed by cancer begins to burn brighter as they share stories in the opening circle. As each brief story is told you can see the bonding starting to happen.

Every one of the hundred-plus cancer retreats we've had at Harmony Hill is unique in its own way, and every individual who attends has a story that is theirs alone. Yet, I see the same alchemy each time we open the retreat in circle. I see people give voice to fears and anger that they've never spoken of before. I see compassion and understanding among strangers who have only just met. I see the love that shines between a husband and wife or between friends. I see the strength and determination that comes from telling our stories and being listened to not just with ears but with hearts. Few things are certain, but the power and magic of the opening circle is something that never fails. ❖

MELODIE PETERSEN:
WHEN CAREGIVERS NEED CARE

As a professional caregiver, Melodie Petersen had reached a point in 2008 where she felt overwhelmed and burned out.

She'd begun working as a nurse in cancer care in 1998, managed the oncology clinic for a year and a half, and then was offered her current position as Cancer Patient Navigator at Providence Regional Cancer System. It was at that point in her career that Melodie felt she desperately needed a sense of renewal.

"My cup was empty," Melodie says, "We nurses give and give and give, and we don't take care of ourselves."

Before transitioning to her new job, she signed up for a health professionals' retreat at Harmony Hill. The retreat was just what she needed – "a breath of fresh air."

It was an emotional three days for Melodie: "I was very tearful from Day One. I needed the reassurance that caregivers need when they're at 'the bottom of the cup.'

"It's amazing how you get so connected so quickly to your retreat group members which, in turn, helps you to reconnect with yourself. Everything about that retreat was so healing – the meditation, walking the peaceful grounds; even something as simple as the hand massages we gave to each other had a profound impact. As we massaged one another's hands, the facilitator spoke loving words aloud for all of us, and it was just, wow, such an act of loving care.

"By the third day, I felt like *I can do this!* To have my feelings and experience acknowledged and validated was so profound it's hard to put into words…."

Melodie's job is to help cancer patients navigate their experience of cancer, to educate and to explain what they can expect, what resources are out there; she helps them make appointments and get to them. If they have no support system, Melodie goes with them to their appointments. A lot of her job, she says, is listening.

And since her personal experience at Harmony Hill, Melodie tells every one of her cancer patients that they need to take advantage of what the Hill has to offer.

"What you gain there – you can't put a price on it. From the time you get out of your car, there's a sense of peacefulness, a sense of awe. It's different than anything or anywhere else I've ever experienced." ❖

> *You gain strength, courage, and confidence by every experience in which you really stop to look fear in the face. You must do the thing which you think you cannot do."*
>
> — ELEANOR ROOSEVELT

CANDIE SCHMITT:
REJOINING THE WORLD

In September 2007, Candie Schmitt was an Early Childhood Special Education Teacher and Director of Elementary School Programs. She was also a busy wife and mother to three grown children.

The final week of that September, Candie went to see her doctor for relief from a persistent headache. The doctor ordered an MRI and made a little joke.

"He said, 'The problem is all in your head,'" she recalls.

"'*Ha ha,*' I laughed.

"Two weeks later I went into Swedish Hospital to have a hemangioma-blastoma (brain tumor) removed. And what was to be a three- to five-day stay in the hospital turned into four months."

The golf-ball sized tumor was located between Candie's brain stem and the cerebellum, and shared blood vessels. During surgery, her vagus nerve was nicked. Doctors and staff didn't think she would survive.

"I lived, but now I walk like the Bride of Frankenstein. I cannot talk. I have a tracheotomy – a tube juts from my neck so that I can breathe, and nutrition is fed to me through tubes to my stomach."

Since the loss of speech, Candie communicates via handwriting and/or her LightWriter, a text-to-voice communication device. (The machine vocalizes what she types.) In person, she expresses herself unambiguously – her lively eyes and vivacious face, her ever-mobile hands, her exuberant spirit articulate so clearly that it's remarkably easy to forget, in the midst of conversation, that Candie is not actually speaking.

She describes her hospital stay: "It was disastrous, in some ways, though the staff was great. I had so many problems – with pneumonia, all the medications, and just being there so long. I was scared and angry. I felt like no one could possibly love me, that they were just putting up with me. My relationship with my husband of 30 years, who had stood by me night and day for months, was unraveling. I'd think, 'Should I have died? Would that have been better for everyone else?' Then I'd think, 'So many people worked so darn hard to save me – I can't disappoint them.'"

Candie went home in a wheelchair at the end of January 2008.

"I had to re-learn how to walk, bit by bit. Physical therapy was a joy for me. I *loved* making progress."

That March, she began using a walker; six months later she started to walk hands-free and improved her gait.

"There's still so much I can't do and probably can never do again. It's so frustrating – you spend your whole life becoming who you are, only to be robbed of that life and having to start over with a different one."

Always a go-getter with an active professional and social life, Candie had never known loneliness and isolation, but she came to know them both all too well when she returned home from the hospital.

"The cure," she says, "is to get out there and do something. Do *something!*

"One of my first victories was indulging in baking therapy," she recollects with a wide smile. "My specialty is blueberry muffins; my neighbors volunteered to be my guinea pigs. Another thing that really helped in the beginning was," as she puts it, "*the stupid TV*. Thank goodness for Ellen Degeneres!"

Her own sense of humor, along with her determination and perseverance, helps keep Candie's morale from flagging, and inspires and delights others. While demonstrating how her LightWriter works, she presses the "joke button" (used only for a laugh with friends) on her keyboard, which declares aloud: *"Ha ha ha! Kiss my patootie!"*

Candie found Harmony Hill while surfing the Internet. Her friend Dixie had also discovered it about the same time – she made a donation to Harmony Hill in Candie's name to encourage Candie to sign up for a cancer retreat. In April 2009, Candie and Steve attended a three-day cancer retreat together at Harmony Hill.

"Above all else, the participants who were there made the retreat an overwhelming success," Candie recalls, "These heroic survivors, willing to share their stories, gave such encouragement to the rest of us.

"A perfect example of the profound effect this sharing had on me was when a woman in our group discussion spoke up and said, 'Cancer is my friend.' My chin must have hit my knees, and I thought, *No way!* But she went on to say what good things have happened to her as a direct result of having had to deal with her health issue. And you know what? She was right! Her statement reminds me to always look for the best in any situation.

"I came away from this retreat feeling that maybe I could rejoin the world. People focused on ability, remarking on the positives. *At Harmony Hill, I felt accepted for who I am now, not who I was in the past.*"

One of Candie's most important goals in 2009 was to attend the graduation ceremonies for "her kids," many of whom she'd known since preschool.

"You could hear a ripple go through the crowd when I came through the door under my own steam," she says. "When the kids stopped by after the ceremony to chit chat, I looked into the matured faces of each of them, and I could see all of those little kids that I knew and loved. I felt so privileged to have played a part in their lives so far. Working with these kids…if I have to die I can go knowing that I made a difference in a lot of lives. Life is amazing." ❧

Living deliberately. For many cancer survivors and many alumni of Harmony Hill, the decision to live deliberately evolves as naturally as their scars heal. Without real effort, a shift occurs in their perspective. For one person, it may be a greater patience for the foibles of others; while for another, it may be a decision to no longer tolerate the prejudice or unkindness of people they once endured quietly. They choose to spend more of their time and energy on thoughts, people, and activities that give their lives meaning. ❧

GREGG SHANK:
THIS IS MY LIFE

Gregg Shank is not a hard man to read. He speaks from the heart, the emotion in his clear blue eyes in complete accord with his words. When asked what Harmony Hill means to him, without hesitation, Gregg says simply, "It probably saved my life."

Harmony Hill is a long way from where Gregg began his life. He grew up in Southern California; he was a child actor in movies and television, spent most his teen years on the beach, and somewhere along the way, Gregg became an addict. Fast forward to 1995: Gregg is now married and has a three-year-old son, Coty, and Gregg is – once again – in rehab, this time in Mason County, Washington. As part of his treatment, he had to pick a place for the community service part of his recovery program. Having been in and out of rehab so many times, Gregg had the desperate feeling that this was his last chance, and he now had a little boy who depended on him. At that point, in one of his *Twelve Step* meetings, Gregg met a man who was also in treatment. His name was Vern.

"My wife was still using. Vern went home with me, saw the situation, and said, 'You'll never get sober in this environment.' I knew he was right, but I didn't know what to do about it. I was going to work at the fairgrounds, but Vern invited me up to Harmony Hill. He was staying there, and he said it was a great place. So I went up to the Hill, met Gretchen, and she agreed that I could do community service up there. Then it was a matter of how to get there…not the easiest thing at that time. I managed to get back and forth a few times, but I knew if I was ever going to get sober, I had to leave my wife. So I went to Harmony Hill with a plastic bag of clothes over my shoulder. Gretchen said I could stay at the cottage and work. I was just taking a leap."

Gregg felt there was something about Harmony Hill, a spiritual feeling that gave him hope.

"There's something there that keeps you going. I didn't know at the time just what it was, but I knew…there was a good chance I could recover there. Folks who were there for cancer retreats were there for a different kind of recovery, but basically they were taking care of themselves, trying to understand themselves and their lives."

And that's what Gregg was trying to do, as he mowed lawns and did odd jobs around the Hill. He vividly recalls one job in particular:

"Gretchen had me clearing dirt under the Lodge so they could put some plumbing in for a new bathroom way at the back of the house. I had to crawl on my belly. There was no room to take a shovel, so I had to dig with these little things, and dig and dig then push the dirt behind me. I could hear people above me in the house; it was so bizarre, and I was thinking about what I was doing. I was moving the earth, pushing it behind me, and I remember thinking to myself, *'This is my life! Get this behind me!'* Harmony Hill brings those kinds of thoughts to mind for me, you know: 'This is my life; this isn't about plumbing. This is just who I am and where I am and what I need to do.' And I just kept digging and digging until I finally had enough room for the plumbing to go through.

"And I was really glad about *that*, too," he adds with a laugh.

Besides the many handyman jobs over the years, Gregg has contributed in other ways to Harmony Hill and to the people who attend the cancer workshops and retreats.

"I don't have cancer, but I was able to sit in on some of the retreats. Sometimes I sat down to dinner with the participants, and I was able to share my story with them. I didn't understand too much about where they were coming from but I felt honored to be there with them and to be able to share with them. Of course, sharing is a big part of recovery – the more you can do it, the better off, the more you're letting go."

Gregg had been at Harmony Hill for a couple years when a new volunteer named Cindy showed up.

"I remember seeing her in the kitchen. Cindy was always in the kitchen, at the window waving. She was struggling with her marriage, and I was separated. I was working on getting full custody of Coty, and got to have him with me on the weekends."

Once both their divorces were behind them, they began spending more time together – Cindy and her daughters with Gregg and his son. Eventually, they became a family; Gregg and Cindy were married on September 3, 2000, at Harmony Hill.

"We just celebrated our tenth anniversary. We watched the video and got to see how the place was back then and to recall all the folks who were there. So many people made that day so special.

"Gretchen has been such a huge blessing. She's always open-armed and she surrounds herself with other people who are also open-armed. So many good and open people - like Jean Moore and Carolyn Olsen.

"Jean is like a big bundle of love. All the FIEs were like that, open-armed and happy to see you.

"And Carolyn: I used to take my son to the restaurant she owned, where I cleaned the kitchen in exchange for meals. Coty would play with people there, Carolyn would talk to friends, and these folks wrote letters of recommendation for my custody hearing. I also worked for Carolyn when she owned a furniture store – until my hips wore out and the doctor made me quit."

"All of them, they're still warm as the day I met them. It's amazing. There was nobody judging me, nobody concerned about who I was, where I came from. It was just, 'You're here. That's good.'"

When he could no longer work at the furniture store, Gregg took college courses (where he was awarded a $500 scholarship) and then got a job with the Shelton Chamber of Commerce, working there for eight years as executive assistant. Through all these changes, he's remained fully involved with Harmony Hill.

"I want to stay connected to the Hill. It's a great place to be; it's always spiritual for me.

"Thinking back on it all now – the two-year custody battle for my son, meeting Gretchen and Carolyn and all – such blessings! I realize that I not only got Coty, but Cindy and the girls and a whole community! *Harmony Hill not only saved my life, it gave me life.*" ❧

GRETCHEN:
THE DAY THE WORLD CHANGED

Like every other American, I have vivid memories of September 11, 2001. I awoke early to find numerous CNN alerts on my computer. Many of our staff were arriving at the same time and we turned the television on. Stunned and disbelieving, we watched the collapse of the twin towers. At the same time, women from the Department of Corrections (DOC) facility at Purdy were arriving to work in the gardens, as they did a few days each week. All of us were drawn like a magnet to the Redwood labyrinth. We formed a large circle around the labyrinth, holding hands, in shock, crying. There must have been twenty or more of us – DOC inmates, corrections officers, Harmony Hill staff, several of our neighbors. We were led in prayer and song by the Purdy DOC women, with each of us participating in our own way from the depths of our hearts and our sorrow. We shared prayers and lamentations of anguish, fear, pain, anger, confusion, forgiveness, and hope. The circle went on for a couple of hours – holding our individual and collective grief, and also cradling us and offering strength. Later, we added large candles to the labyrinth and kept them burning for days. For months after 9/11, many of our staff and the Purdy DOC women made daily sojourns to the labyrinth to meditate and offer prayers for healing.

During those painful weeks after the tragedy we felt particularly blessed to be in the healing environment of Harmony Hill. Many people were drawn to the Hill. People we knew, and people we had never seen before, came and asked permission to wander the grounds, to sit in the gardens, or to walk the labyrinth. They, like us, found comfort in the tranquility and beauty of Harmony Hill. Indeed, the unity, accord, and peacefulness of our name and our nature proved consolation to so many. There have been other horrific disasters since 9/11, and there undoubtedly will be more. I find comfort in knowing that the Hill not only provides a place of respite and sanctuary – however brief – it also holds and sends forth the intentions of so many to promote peace and compassion, and to recognize our inevitable and indestructible interconnectedness. ❧

Many people have likened the feeling they had when they received their cancer diagnosis to the emotions they felt on 9/11. They cite feelings of numbness, disbelief, helplessness, and a certainty that the world would never be the same. Said one cancer survivor, "Before my cancer diagnosis, I felt impervious. Suddenly – in the space of just moments – I knew that I was not. I felt frightened and very vulnerable."

Just as 9/11 was a lesson of both unspeakable evil and unparalleled acts of kindness, cancer is also a lesson in polarities. It's a dance of fear and hope, anger and gratitude, vulnerability and strength. It's a dance commenced without knowing the steps, but knowing that each step taken leads to the next, and then the next, and – for a time – that is enough. ❧

CHAPTER FOUR:
Letting go – the gift of vulnerability

"When I was diagnosed with cancer, one of the things I dealt with was the changes to my body. The removal of parts of my body I had previously thought I could never let go of.... I may have been beaten down by the cancer, but I did rise – taller, stronger, more vibrantly alive than before."
— RUTHANN MCCANN, HARMONY HILL ALUMNA

Accepting *what is* is not something that comes easily to most of us. Especially when "what is" is not what we had planned for ourselves. There's an old saying, "If you want to make God laugh, just tell him your plans." It's easy to accept all the good things that come to us unannounced and unplanned – surely we deserved them. It's not so easy to accept the losses, the disappointments, or the unwelcome diagnosis – what did we do to deserve *this*?

Acceptance is not defeat and surrender is not submission. Accepting is often the first step in opening ourselves to unseen options, and surrender might be the first step in trusting that the universe might hold us if we release our tight grip and *let go*. Many of us are raised to be self-sufficient, rewarded for being stoic and for not showing our weakness. Suddenly, we're thrust into a situation that requires us to depend on the advice and treatment of unknown medical professionals, and to rely on family, friends, and even strangers to help us get through the day.

Many people who have journeyed through cancer have not only learned these lessons but embraced them as the opening to deeper understanding of themselves and their connectedness in the world. Words like "vulnerability" and "need" lose their sting and become badges of strength and incentives for perceiving the world in new ways and experiencing gratitude at a new level. ❧

GRETCHEN:
FATEFUL JOURNEY

In November of 2001, I traveled to New York City to support three runners who were participating in the city's famed marathon to raise funds for Harmony Hill. It was a particularly poignant year – more than two million people were there to cheer on the runners, many of whom were running in memory of loved ones who had died just weeks before in the attacks on the World Trade Center. While I was there, I witnessed the overwhelming devastation of 9/11 and the scars it had left on New York and its residents. I also saw the amazing outpouring of love and compassion that lifted the city above the destruction and inspired the world.

On the flight home, while pondering the extremes of kindness and cruelty that we humans are capable of, I noticed a persistent pain in my left groin, and swelling in my left leg. It was just two weeks later that I was diagnosed with non-Hodgkin's lymphoma. Suddenly, I was no longer just a witness and facilitator for those on a cancer journey. I had joined them on the journey, and, as I knew from witnessing so many journeys, life would never be the same.

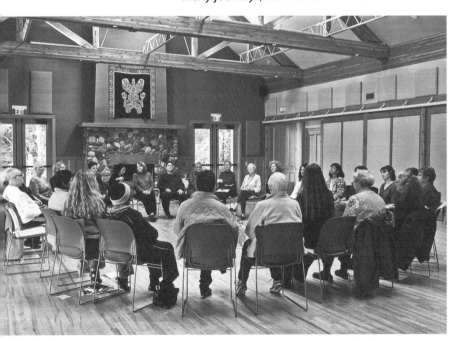

A "sacred circle" group session during a cancer retreat in the Elmer and Katharine Nordstrom Great Hall.

Like every participant in Harmony Hill's cancer retreats, I have my own stories of treatment: placement of a port for chemotherapy, the chemo, losing my hair, my eyebrows, and my eyelashes (this last was the hardest – I felt so naked!), the weariness, and the fears…. And I have stories of the immense expressions of love and support from so many friends, family, colleagues, and acquaintances. I gained a new perspective on what life really means and saw with new eyes the power of deeply shared experience. ❖

JUDY DUNCAN:
UNFOLDING VULNERABILITY...
BREATHING IN HOPE

Judy Duncan attended Harmony Hill's three-day cancer retreat in February 2008. After treatment for breast cancer in 1996, she was cancer-free for five years before being diagnosed again with breast cancer in 2006. This cancer had metastasized and Judy's new normal became living with Stage 4 incurable cancer. Four surgeries and many rounds of chemo and radiation later, she remains an indomitable spirit.

Judy grew up with a positive outlook. She chose the kangaroo as her totem, it being the only animal that is incapable of moving backward.

"I look back only to learn the lessons, then I keep moving forward."

For her, the glass is more than half-full, or even full – it's *overflowing*. She shares that outlook with friends, family, fellow travelers on the cancer journey, and her medical teams. Before each surgery, Judy has led her surgical team in a rousing rendition of the "Happy Cell Song," an upbeat song that she sings daily and teaches to others.

Judy describes herself as a typical Type A personality. After her diagnosis, she vowed to be "the best cancer patient, the best chemo patient that ever was." She was determined that no one would ever see her weak, or depressed, or needy.

Sometimes the universe has other plans for us. Of the many gifts Judy received at Harmony Hill, the experience of a safe place to be vulnerable turned out to be paramount. It was the safety of the group sessions and the skilled and gentle guidance of the facilitators that allowed her to feel her own vulnerability and to let others see that vulnerability in her. With new clarity she became aware that the vulnerability that she witnessed unfolding was not a weakness, but a strength. She was able to honor previously denied feelings of vulnerability, frailty, or sadness, seeing them now as making her whole. Instead of denying parts of who she was, she embraced it all.

"Harmony Hill opened me up.

"After all those years of being the person others came to for support, the one whom others asked for help, I've given myself permission to do the same. If I'm down, I can pick up the phone and call a friend, I can ask for help. And there's a gift in that for my friends and family. They don't feel shut out. They have something precious to share with me.

"I went to Harmony Hill holding my breath. But I ended up breathing out my fears and breathing in hope… I've been doing so ever since."

At the suggestion of one of the Harmony Hill facilitators, Judy has embarked on a new adventure with her positive approach to life. She is being trained in laughter therapy – instruction in the physical aspects of laughter: how to laugh deeply to release stress and promote healing.

"If you simulate laughter, you stimulate laughter," Judy says. Shortly, she will become a certified laughter therapy leader and her hope is to work with cancer groups to share the power and magic of laughter. "This, too, is a gift I received from Harmony Hill that has provided me a purpose and set my priorities for the time I have left. I'm living the life I want to live. What you put out does come back to you tenfold."

Judy declares proudly, "I love life!" and she's living it to its full depth and breadth…and showing others how to do so, as well.

"Harmony Hill was life-changing. It allowed me to feel and honor everything that I was feeling and everything that I am. Instead of denying or trying to hide my sadness or vulnerability, I could own them and become whole. It was freeing." ❖

> "We are all here for a spell. Get all the good laughs you can."
> – WILL ROGERS

GRETCHEN:
THE JOURNEY OF A THOUSAND STEPS…

My own cancer journey gave me an even greater appreciation and admiration for the individuals who attend our cancer retreats, for their courage and their honesty. The ability to be open and compassionate in the face of something so big – so threatening – speaks volumes for the human spirit. This is true not just for those dealing with a cancer diagnosis, but also for their families and loved ones who provide support and acceptance in the face of their own fears and uncertainty.

I started a six-month course of chemotherapy – CHOP, which I renamed "Chopin," and Rituxan – in late November 2001. There is a point in between chemo treatments that medical professionals call the "nadir" – it's the lowest physiological point when blood counts are low and energy depleted. I'd always been blessed with boundless energy, so nadirs became a great teacher for me. I learned to appreciate each moment as it occurred, and to prioritize my activities. What was really important to me? And what could I let go of? Was this worry, or this frustration, worthy of giving my limited energy to?

I was blessed with an excellent medical team of both conventional and integrative members. One example of a complementary therapy that I benefited from enormously was listening to a guided imagery CD developed for people with cancer by psychotherapist Belleruth Naparstek. She has produced numerous CDs for a wide variety of medical diagnoses and wellness issues. Many people find them extremely beneficial. I was particularly drawn to one affirmation that acknowledged the lessons cancer teaches us: *"Thank you for teaching me to stop and listen. Thank you for reminding me of what is truly important. You can go now."*

A few weeks earlier, while waiting for my diagnosis, I shared what was happening during a women's leadership workshop and support circle I attended at the Whidbey Institute. Someone in the group asked me what my favorite color was and I said "blue-green." They told me whenever I was concerned or frightened, I should envision myself being wrapped by them in a soft, warm, blue-green blanket. That image gave me a sense of comfort and confidence that accompanied me throughout my medical journey … and still does today.

I adapted another affirmation from Belleruth Naparstek: "I can look inside my body and see a powerful blue-green wave of pure healing washing through it from head to toe, clearing out any unwanted debris and taking it out with the tide." Blue-green images started showing up everywhere, from the lab coat of my doctor's nurse, to the candles we lit on the fireplace mantle. I felt surrounded by healing energy.

I was also moved beyond words by the enormous outpouring of love and support I received from friends, family, and colleagues, both near and far. I understood completely what so many of our cancer retreat alumni meant when they said they felt like they were "being held totally and lovingly." It's a feeling that really defies description, but warms the heart and fills one with a deep and absolute sense of wellbeing.

A physician friend – a psychiatrist and internist who specializes in stress reduction – sent me information about humor therapy. He noted that "cancer cells reputedly cannot stand laughter." He attached pages of comical snippets which were the answers sixth-graders gave to a history test. I hadn't laughed so hard in years. While I can't definitively prove the efficacy of humor therapy, it became one of the tools for my journey. I recommend it highly!

The lessons of cancer were vast, as was my sense of gratitude. I also came to fully understand a term we regularly used in our cancer retreats: "new normal." For a person dealing with cancer, new normal describes how life has changed – in ways both welcome and uninvited. New normal also encompasses living with the uncertainty of cancer – diagnosis, treatment, outcomes, recurrences….

I've mentioned before that at the beginning of each retreat I had always shared with participants a favorite quote: *Life is not about waiting for the storms to pass, it's about learning to dance in the rain.* Now, when I share that saying, it's more than an inspiring notion, it's a way of living. We do a lot of dancing in the rain around here! ❖

> "Gratitude unlocks the fullness of life. It turns what we have into enough, and more. It turns denial into acceptance, chaos to order, confusion to clarity. It can turn a meal into a feast, a house into a home, a stranger into a friend. Gratitude makes sense of our past, brings peace for today, and creates a vision for tomorrow."
>
> – MELODY BEATTIE

BARBARA OSWALD:
COURAGE TO BE AUTHENTIC

Just as Barbara Oswald never allowed the fact that she is blind to define her, neither did she allow her cancer diagnosis in 2006 to define or limit her. The day she was told she had breast cancer, Barbara and a friend had planned to take their first kayaking lesson. Barbara saw no reason to change their plans.

"Hey, I've got cancer; what have I got to lose?" she reminded herself as the instructor attempted to describe in words for her what he usually demonstrated for sighted students: how to flip the kayak, climb out while submerged upside-down, and then turn the boat over and climb back in.

"I can do this," said Barbara, and then she did.

She faces most things with similar determination, yet she acknowledges that there are many things she has not been able to do because of her blindness: "Hop in a car and drive my daughter to ballet class or soccer practice, or be the jitney-bus mom." But people are surprised by how many things she does. Barbara is an accomplished artist – a painter and photographer. Her photographs are stunning scenes from nature, perfectly composed and highly evocative.

"I don't take pictures of what I see," she says, "I take pictures of what feels like the right thing. It's not until later that I know exactly what I'm photographing."

She also runs a cozy bed-and-breakfast in Seattle's Mt. Baker area, near the shores of Lake Washington. Casa de Esperanza (House of Hope) is a 1930's art deco hacienda entered through a peaceful courtyard garden. It also houses a gallery of art by artists with disabilities. The living room walls at Casa de Esperanza are hung with paintings and photographs depicting serene landscapes, seascapes, colorful still-lifes, and human figures. The mantelpiece showcases intricate scrimshaw carvings. All are by artists who are visually impaired. One would never guess it – not in a hundred years.

While Barbara welcomes any guest to Casa de Esperanza, she particularly relishes the opportunity to host individuals who are visiting Seattle for cancer treatment. She remembers being alone for much of her own cancer journey and wants to offer others a place of comfort and healing. Close to downtown Seattle and its many medical facilities, Casa de Esperanza offers a comfortable bed, healthy organic food – much of which Barbara grows herself in her welcoming "survivors' garden" – and a safe, comfortable place from which to navigate the cancer journey.

In some ways, Barbara says, being blind prepared her for dealing with cancer.

"Because there's a limit to what you can do, you have a choice. You can either rail against your limitations or you can say, 'Okay, how can I be whole in the face of this?' Blindness equipped me with the patience I needed when cancer knocked me flat.

"Because I learned long ago to navigate a world I couldn't see and to deal with obstacles that appeared in front of me suddenly, I carried with me on my cancer journey a sense that I could maneuver in this new environment despite any rocks or potholes that would inevitably be placed in my path. I was lucky to already have the tools that most people have to learn on the fly after a cancer diagnosis."

Barbara attended Harmony Hill's three-day cancer retreat in March of 2007.

"I remember being tremendously depleted from the cancer treatment. I was really tired and yet unable to sleep. I was living alone and the nights were so long. I just wanted some human beings to be around. That's what I was looking forward to at Harmony Hill…I was tired of being by myself. I thought, 'Oh, goody, I'm going to camp! – Cancer Camp'

"And just like camp, there were so many activities and I wanted to do everything. I pretty much did, too! What I loved most were the singing bowls. They were magical, incredible…and they made such a beautiful sound. They were said to have healing properties. I couldn't get enough of them."

Barbara's career has been spent working in the disability field. She is aware, both as an advocate and as a blind person, that people's differences are not always seen or understood by others, and that their needs are not always recognized by those around them.

"Each of us who came to Harmony Hill had a disability, whether it was our cancer, our vulnerability in the face of it, or perhaps it had nothing to do with cancer, but related to another injury or loss we may have been carrying around for years. Most of us needed accommodation of some sort, many not as evident as my own. I wondered if the people at Harmony Hill were prepared to deal with our differences and our many, varied needs.

"They did so magnificently! Each of us was accepted just as we were and we were given just what we needed. I was surprised that there was a vessel to hold all of the hurt, not just the cancer."

"When I was going through treatment," Barbara recalls, "I was very frightened at the prospect of radiation. It terrified me. I refused it. My surgeon told me that her work would be wasted if I didn't follow through on the radiation, but still I hesitated. A friend asked me, 'What if you saw it as something beautiful, as something that would heal you?' Together, we came up with the idea of a permeable love shield that would direct the love and counteract the negative aspects of radiation. I decided I needed a shield of pink roses and asked my friends to send pink rose images to remind me to let the love in, let the pain go, and acknowledge the beauty." Barbara made a montage of the cards, pictures and encouraging messages her friends sent. In the center of the shield, amidst an abundance of pink blossoms, are the words, *"If you want what you've never had, then do what you've never done."*

"After Harmony Hill, I knew I wanted to offer some sort of love shield for people on their own cancer journeys. That's when I envisioned this house as a B&B for people dealing with cancer treatment. Casa de Esperanza is a place of comfort and safety. It's a place where they don't have to be alone."

Throughout her cancer journey, Barbara has been reminded of the rewards of being authentic and allowing herself to be vulnerable. She recalls her appointment with her radiologist a few weeks into her radiation treatment. "How do you feel?" he asked.

"Do I say what is real or make nice talk?" That was the question she faced. "I told him, 'I feel like a frightened two-year-old.' That halted him. He asked me 'What do you need?' 'I need a hug,' I told him.

"He stopped everything else and gave me the biggest hug. It was just what I needed. Then he turned to his nurse and dictated a prescription that I was to be given a hug each time I came in for radiation treatment. Those hugs helped me through. What if I had been afraid to admit how frightened I was, afraid to tell him what I needed? We need to allow ourselves to be vulnerable."

Barbara frequently refers to her cancer experience as a journey: "Cancer was really hard, but there were moments of pure beauty and delight. It was a dance with many movements and steps, some I wouldn't trade for the world because I'm a much more whole human being now."

One of the blessings of cancer is what Barbara refers to as the "spirituality of diminishment."

"We must be willing to get rid of the life we've planned, so as to have the life that is waiting for us."
– JOSEPH CAMPBELL

"It's something I thought I knew a lot about due to my lifelong alliance with blindness. But the experience of cancer called me to examine this spirituality from a totally different place. Being able to accept what is, what is in the moment, what is now, not what was yesterday, or last week, or a year ago. As Americans, we are taught how to hold on, how to collect things; we're told not to let go. But there is something wondrous about learning how to let go and about learning how to be where you are when you're there, be present in the moment.

"It was an incredible blessing to learn how to let go. Cancer gave that to me, and Harmony Hill reinforced it. The other big gift I got from Harmony Hill was the reaffirmation in me to be authentic, to say what I feel and to ask for what I need. These are precious gifts!" ❖

Letting go and acceptance are two sides of the same door. Both are simple concepts; both are difficult practices. And both are necessary steps to three major portals of healing: courage, compassion and connection.

When faced with fear, uncertainty and loss, the natural tendency for most people is to clasp the reins of control, to hold on tighter than ever to the known, and to struggle to regain our footing on the well-worn, familiar path.

It's a great feat of spirit to let go *with all our might* and allow the wisdom of insecurity to guide us through the unknown.

In order to feel secure, most people have formed the habit of looking behind and ahead, which makes it difficult to be fully present in the here and now. By letting go of the illusion of everlasting security, we're able to experience the freedom of the Zen concept of "beginner's mind." Letting go allows us to stay open to new possibilities, and to re-enter the flow of life. ❖

NORMA SCHUITEMAN:
WHAT THE HUMAN SPIRIT IS CAPABLE OF

The first time Norma Schuiteman went to Harmony Hill it was to conduct a site visit, a walk-through of the new Creekside building; just part of doing her job in grant fund requests at the Community Foundation.

She didn't meet Gretchen Schodde until a later date, when Norma, a trained Executive Coach, was leading a program for non-profits.

"I guess Gretchen was impressed with the program and with me because she invited me to Harmony Hill," says Norma, "and somewhere along the line I became a housemother." Although Norma's a registered nurse, she hadn't practiced for a long time and wasn't sure she was up to the job. "But Gretchen said, 'Yes! You can do it, Norma.'"

Norma put her name on the list of housemothers, to fill in for emergencies. She went to her first retreat with fear and trembling ("too many opportunities to screw up," she remembers thinking.) And now she always has her name on the list and is a housemom at least once a year.

What hooked her? "I was struck by what could happen in the course of three days. The change was so significant, says Norma, that "I was touched to my pith about the human spirit, what it's capable of." She discovered that Harmony Hill is a place where one could feel not just safe but surrounded by beauty of many kinds, to find strength they didn't know they had or that had been buried.

"I felt better each time I served as a housemom," Norma recalls. "I went to at least one session each time, and no matter what the session was like, I always came away better than when I was before."

Over time, Norma has come to value the uniqueness of Harmony Hill. When asked what she thinks makes Harmony Hill so unique, Norma hesitates only a moment.

"Well, it sounds trite but it's so…*organic*. Goodness emerges effortlessly because it's inherently good. It offers safety, serenity, and tranquility in a professional (medically and holistically) environment. The place really demonstrates the power of a vision."

The last time Norma was a housemother she witnessed the power of that vision in action.

"When this particular cancer-retreat group arrived (and they all have their distinct group dynamics), I could see there was *some* openness, but a great deal of pain and tightness. They went around the circle, talked a little, and went to dinner. Afterwards, they gathered for a meeting and were really closed and inner-focused. I didn't meet with the group again until the following evening, when it was time for hand and foot massages. I wasn't sure what to expect. At the end of one and a half, maybe two hours, people were laughing! They were so noisy, having so much fun. I was just wiped out! They had come in around two or three o'clock the previous afternoon and by nine o'clock the second night, there was this metamorphosis that, to me, typifies the sanctity of Harmony Hill. It was simply profound." ✢

> **"**Choose life – only that and always, and at whatever risk. To let life leak out, to let it wear away by the mere passage of time, to withhold giving it and spreading it is to choose nothing."
>
> – SR. HELEN KELLEY

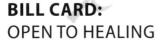

BILL CARD:
OPEN TO HEALING

Bill Card was 30 years old in 2000, when he was diagnosed with cancer.

"I was the typical stubborn male," he says, "I was determined to tough it out, to beat it, to get on with life."

And, in a way, he did. Bill went through treatment, including potent rounds of chemotherapy. He survived the cancer, but his marriage didn't. Bill and his wife grew apart during those years of treatment and recovery. She left him in 2005, but not before leaving a brochure about Harmony Hill on his desk. "I thought I had beaten the cancer, I was past it. Why would I need this? But then, when my wife left, I fell apart. Those five years were such an intense and emotional time, and I just kept trying to push everything under the rug."

When he opened his newspaper to an article about Harmony Hill, Bill finally acknowledged that maybe it was a sign.

"Living in Shelton, I'm not that far away, so I rode my bike over to Harmony Hill to see what it was all about. The second I got on the grounds, I had this intense sense of healing. I realized I should have come here a long time ago. Gretchen was there and I talked with her and a few other people there about what was going on with me. They said they could get me into a one-day workshop in a few weeks and put me on the waiting list for the three-day retreat. It felt like the right place to be, the right thing to do.

"Thanks to Cindy Shank's diligent efforts, I was able to go to the 'Tools' workshop that fall and then to attend the three-day in January of 2006. That was such an amazing experience. Most of all, I remember the feelings of peace and safety I had there. My room was in the Creekside building and it was so peaceful. It felt like I was among people who were going through the same journey I was. They understood what it was like, and it was safe – really safe – to open myself up completely.

"The past five years had been so intense and emotional, yet I had denied so much of what I was feeling. At Harmony Hill, it was safe to let it all out, to share things I'd never shared before – my fears, my anger, my loneliness, my survivor's guilt. It was okay to cry. And there was no judgment, just acceptance and understanding.

"There were so many things that I'd been feeling that I couldn't share with anyone, that no one else understood, but here, *everyone* understood. Everyone in that room was connected by that understanding.

"It was an amazing experience to spend three days just being loved and nurtured, being watched over. And the fact that it was free makes it even more remarkable. You can be there without worrying about the cost. So many people who need Harmony Hill wouldn't be able to go there if they had to bear the financial burden themselves."

Bill was introduced to yoga at Harmony Hill.

"I'd never done it before. I was paired with a woman for an exercise that we did back to back, and at one point we could feel each other's hearts beating through our backs – it was amazing to share that feeling of our life-forces pulsing together!"

A baker by profession, Bill has immense appreciation for the kitchen at Harmony Hill, and the care that went into the meals they were served.

"It was top-notch; it was beyond good. They have a beautiful kitchen garden where they grow so much of what they serve there. There's just so much love. It's evident in everything they do."

Those three days were just the start, explains Bill. "I've said many times that Harmony Hill saved my life. There are so many tools they give you to take home. I went there a mess spiritually and mentally, and I came away with an inner peace that remains with me. I came out of it so blessed!"

"*I remember starting to beat myself up, 'Why didn't I come here before? Why? Why? Why?' But during the retreat someone told me, 'You get here when it's your time and now is your time.' How true that is. I was ready to be opened up, and I was.*" ❖

MIM COLLINS:
EBB AND FLOW

In 2009, Mim Collins was a year into Cardio and Kinesis training at Vera, a women's gym *par excellence*. It was a wonderful, enriching, playful time for her; the group enjoyed a wide variety of fun things together. Above all, Mim savored the spirit of community she found there.

> **"**I do not believe that sheer suffering teaches. If suffering alone taught, all the world would be wise, since everyone suffers. To suffering must be added mourning, understanding, patience, love, openness, and the willingness to remain vulnerable.**"**
>
> – ANNE MORROW LINDBERGH

When her belly began getting "round and fussy," she stepped back from the training, and began eating only soft grains and steamed vegetables. Mim knows a good deal about nutrition. Though she's a psychotherapist by profession, she also had one of the first natural food cooking schools in the Pacific Northwest.

"I thought I was having a stress reaction because my closest friend was hit with early Alzheimer's in 2009, and I was doing everything possible for her. So by June, when my husband and I went to Alaska, I was ready to take a break. Unfortunately, my stomach didn't take a break."

One day, shortly after they'd returned home from their trip, Mim's husband hugged her and commented that her stomach was not only round, it was also quite firm. So Mim got on the phone to her doctor.

"Just 11 months prior, my doctor had suggested we add a CA125 to my regular lab tests – that's the determinate for any cancer cells in the body. I now urge everyone to get one. It's not conclusive, but it's a good indicator. Normal is 0 – 35 and I was in the low normal less than a year before, now it was over 300.

"I knew about cancer – two of my aunts had it, my mother died of uterine cancer, and my son's father died of cancer. So I had an intimate relationship with the disease, but I never believed I'd get it.

"The diagnostic process was three steps: the CA125, an ultrasound, and then a CAT scan, which was conclusive: it was primary peritoneal cancer, in the area below my navel."

Mim went to Cancer Care Alliance and had the good fortune to be assigned a doctor famous for her research in gynecologic cancers. Eight days after her diagnosis, Mim's doctor informed her of the necessary treatment – a total hysterectomy followed by chemotherapy.

"On the 4th of July, there was a circle of *so* many women in my yard! All come to bless and prepare and send me on my way to surgery. They handed me a yellow packet that was full of song and dance and blessings and good will, and a whole care system was set up for me!"

Mim had her hysterectomy and was in the hospital for three days. Then it was time for chemotherapy.

"The prospect of the infusion of highly toxic chemicals into my body was very frightening. At the hospital I asked everyone to leave me alone because I began to find that the quiet of working with this medicine was important. I thought of it as an elixir of magic and wellness. The night before, a woman from the Native American tradition came to visit, and she had made this basket for me; in it were some shells. She had learned that you can work with chemo like the ocean. I took that basket to every treatment. And while I was receiving the infusion I worked with that image: what I needed was coming in and what I needed to release was going out. At the end of this day that I had so feared, I was driven home by family and when I got out of car, I said, 'I'm hungry, let's call the neighbors and see what's for dinner!'"

Every three weeks, another all-day chemo treatment. Mim had had two treatments by the time her birthday came around in September.

"That evening my husband presented me with a gift, asked me to come and sit down with him and proceeded to tell me that in January he would be filing for divorce. This came so completely out of the blue from my husband and was so out of character, it *frightened* me. I never saw it coming. I went into trauma and shock, thinking, 'Well, *now* what am I going to do?'"

Mim called a friend and went to her home for a few days. With that "great sisterly support," she began to problem-solve. She got a legal separation and her husband moved out of the house.

"It was winter, I was going through chemo, and I began to feel a bit frightened being alone at home. And then, without really a plan around that, a succession of women would come to my home. Sometimes we didn't even see each other, they would just come – I would be in bed at 7:30, and they knew where the guest room was. It was *such* tremendous support."

Mim's last scheduled day of chemo was on December 15, 2009, and she was beginning to see the light at the end of the tunnel. She celebrated with a trip to sunny California with her sister, then returned to work on December 28. That night, she had the worst stomach pains she'd ever experienced and had to go into the hospital. It turned out that a small bowel obstruction had been caused by adhesions from her first operation. It became clear that another surgery was necessary. That hospital stay was twelve days.

Her doctor performed fifteen biopsies – fourteen were benign, one showed a residual cancer.

"My doctor told me to go home and rest up for a month and then we'd start chemo again. She said, 'Get your support circle, then come and listen to your treatment options.'"

Presented with a drug that was the wave of the future – PARP inhibitor – Mim opted to be part of an initial study for the drug. She began this round of chemo toward the end of February.

Over the course of the six-month treatment, Mim began to feel a draw to do a "group cancer experience," so she went to Harmony Hill.

"It was my first time being with a group of cancer patients. My roommate came from Florida, and she had a very complicated cancer. We became very supportive of each other. She would leave her light on, and just sort of sit and sleep; she didn't move all night. I had hit a stretch of sleep-challenge during treatment, and I just would watch her sleeping so soundly. There's something about knowing that a sister on the journey is sleeping deeply all night; it was such an unexpected delight.

"And there was another great gift for me, personally. Part of the weekend was spent doing yoga and dancing. I'm a dancer and I hadn't been dancing all this time. At the end of the retreat, when we were saying our good-byes to one another, I came to the dance facilitator and just started sobbing – because I had been *reawakened*. We were given so much permission to delve into what we needed to delve into; and when you're going through such invasive, intensive treatment, that is a tremendous gift, a very gracious gift."

At the end of her last round of chemotherapy, Mim was thoroughly tested, and the tests were conclusive.

"My doctor looked me in the eye and told me I was *in remission, cancer free, a survivor* – all those words that you wonder when and if you'll hear. That was July 6, 2010, exactly 365 days after my first surgery.

"I had planned a potlatch party that evening, and there were about thirty women again on my lawn. I made the main dish, this delicious spinach pie from Harmony Hill, which everyone loved. I'd set out chairs, but nobody sat in them. We all sat together on the ground… in a circle." ❖

"How can you follow the course of your life if you do not let it flow?"

– LAO-TZU

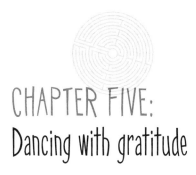

CHAPTER FIVE:
Dancing with gratitude

"I learned that cancer for me has been a gift. I am OK. I can be in control of my health and body. I am empowered now to take charge of my life and where it is going. I am now doing what I always thought about doing in the future." – MARGE PUTNAM, 2003 HARMONY HILL ALUMNA

"Gratitude" and "cancer" are words that aren't often paired. But gratitude has been a constant throughout Harmony Hill's 25-year history, and also a word that one hears frequently in conversations with alumni of the Hill's cancer retreat programs.

It may seem preposterous to call cancer a gift, but many people are surprised to find they do call it just that. A gift. In his wonderful book, *Chasing Daylight*, Eugene O'Kelley, facing advanced and inoperable brain cancer, expresses his gratitude for "the journey that allowed me to experience what was there all along but had been hidden thanks to the distractions of the world." And for those lucky enough to survive the cancer, whether it's for a few months, a few years, or for many decades, they often retain that new awareness, that heightened sense of aliveness. The door that opened stays open. ❖

RICARDO GOMEZ:
BREATHE AND CELEBRATE

So many lessons. Many of them painful, many of them beautiful. When Ricardo Gomez reflects back on nearly five years of cancer, caregiving, grief, and new beginnings, he sees so many lessons.

"Maybe I just need to remember the simplest thing: breathe in, breathe out, repeat. One step at a time. One day at a time."

Ricardo has a deep and multi-faceted connection to Harmony Hill. He accompanied his late wife, Claudia, there twice following her diagnosis of advanced-stage ovarian cancer. Additionally, he attended a three-day caregiver retreat while caring for Claudia, and another shortly after her death. A year later, he was there for a retreat during his own treatment for thyroid cancer. And, finally, on a sun-drenched Fourth of July in 2010, he was at Harmony Hill for a very different reason - to celebrate with friends and family his marriage to Mary.

"It's a place of transformation," he says, "Not just for dealing with the challenges of cancer, but also for new beginnings. A place becomes different depending on the lens you use to look at it.

"Harmony Hill helped me deal with my wife's cancer better, and with my role as her caregiver. Later, it helped me deal with my own cancer. It put me in touch with many forms of wellness and self-care, practices that I carry forward today. And still later, its beauty and energy inaugurated a new chapter of my life, a new relationship."

Most striking to Ricardo was what one retreat facilitator, Cobie, described as the "accelerated authenticity" that happens at Harmony Hill.

"You get together a group of strangers and very quickly you get into a profound and authentic state of sharing through a quickened process. Harmony Hill has such a potent energy. What happens there is powerful."

In conversations with other caregivers, Ricardo found ways to care for himself amidst the stress of caring for his wife.

"As caregivers, we are almost always focused on the other person, on our role as a caregiver. We need to be reminded to take care of ourselves. We also need to recognize that there are things we cannot fix, but we can learn to deal with them better. Harmony Hill was a place to plug in and recharge my batteries; it was a space to decompress and find a sort of peace."

Many people have said that a lesson of cancer, and of Harmony Hill, is learning to accept help, and learning to ask for help. Ricardo notes that it was a lesson he, too, learned.

"Asking for help and accepting the help of others is hard for most of us. The real lesson, though, is learning to accept help the way it comes and being gracious no matter what. When I took over laundry duty, Claudia had a hard time surrendering to the fact that I didn't do it just as she had. And when friends brought us meals, we learned to accept them gratefully, even if they weren't something that we would have cooked for ourselves. People help for their own reasons, and in their own ways, and accepting their help in the ways they want to give it was a tremendous lesson: *This is something given to us by somebody in the universe, and we can be grateful for their gifts, and for life's gifts.*"

Ricardo continues, "The 'undergraduate' lesson was learning to ask for help, and having to accept that you can't do it alone. But the 'graduate school' lesson was learning to accept the help in whatever way it came."

When Ricardo received his own cancer diagnosis less than a year after Claudia's death, friends asked, "Why this? Why now?" Ricardo found he was strangely at peace. He noted in his blog, "It is what it is, and there is no reason. I may not like it, but I can love it for what it shows me, teaches me, allows me to learn. I don't like it, but I can learn to love it – one more experience that gives meaning to my life."

When Claudia was first diagnosed, Ricardo started the blog. Originally, it was intended to keep family and friends informed of her progress and treatment, saving the family many phone calls and e-mails during stressful times. Ricardo discovered that the writing was therapeutic for him, it helped him find meaning and gave him a way to pause and explore life as it was unfolding. Friends and family found it inspirational and urged him to consider publishing it. Late in 2010, *Breathe and Celebrate* was published, chronicling the five years during which Ricardo, Claudia, and their family dealt with her illness, then the grief of her loss, the challenge of Ricardo's own cancer diagnosis, a new relationship, and, finally, marriage to Mary at Harmony Hill. The book is a moving account of love, family, friendship, resilience, gratitude, and – as the title suggests – living in the present and finding reasons for celebration wherever and whenever possible. Ricardo has directed that all proceeds from the sale of the book go to Harmony Hill.

Publishing the book symbolized turning the page to the next stage of Ricardo's life. "I don't know if others will be interested in our story, or in the learning that came through it for me. It is out there, like a paper boat on a stream or a message in a bottle; the rest is not in my control. If it can help someone, or help Harmony Hill, then I am doubly blessed."

Reflecting on the blessing of finding Mary amidst so much personal challenge, Ricardo recalls, "Our wedding at Harmony Hill was a two-and-a-half day celebration. Close family and friends came and stayed with us the day before, and then more friends joined us on the day of the wedding. In all, there must have been a hundred or so. Everyone commented on the beauty of the place, the peacefulness and friendliness. And the food was tremendous – everyone loved it. An energy of wellness surrounded us.... We were married outdoors, right in the middle of the labyrinth. It's a fantastic place to have a wedding!"

"Harmony Hill offers a support that goes into great depth. Of necessity, it reaches only a small number of people at each retreat, but those people are touched in a profound and transformational way. That is a very valuable and precious thing...it makes a huge difference. There are other programs that might reach more people, but they often skim the surface. Harmony Hill goes deep." ❧

"If the only prayer you say in your entire life is 'thank you,' that would suffice."

– MEISTER ECKHART

Sometimes it's easier to give than to receive. Most of us are brought up to be self-sufficient, rewarded for being strong and capable. Sometimes, though, even the most capable among us need help, and that can be hard for us to admit or accept. The ability to ask for help when we need it becomes a strength, not a weakness. It helps immensely to know that generally our friends, our family, often even acquaintances and perfect strangers are eager to assist. It feels good to be needed, it feels good to see that we can make a difference in someone's life. It is not a one-sided relationship, for in giving the giver also receives much. It's one of those lessons we learn over and over.

Many who attend Harmony Hill retreats comment on how strange it felt at first to have so many people – most of them strangers – so eager to support them and to provide for them in unexpected ways. Whether it was assistance with an activity, a kind word, a hug, a foot massage, a delicious meal, or that rarest of things: acceptance without judgment – attendees note that a shift occurred when they were able to accept these gifts. They didn't feel so alone, they felt valued, and they felt whole. With a deeper awareness of the interconnectedness of everything, they also found that they were more able to extend their own gifts to others.

Maybe this is because Harmony Hill exemplifies the difference between "helping" and "serving" that Rachel Remen has eloquently discussed. Dr. Remen notes that "Service is a relationship between equals," while "helping incurs debt.

"When you help someone, they owe you. But serving, like healing, is mutual. There is no debt. I am as served as the person I am serving. When I help I have a feeling of satisfaction. When I serve I have a feeling of gratitude. These are very different things.

"When I help," says Remen, "I am very aware of my own strength. But we don't serve with our strength; we serve with ourselves. We draw from all of our experiences. Our limitations serve, our wounds serve, even our darkness can serve. The wholeness in us serves the wholeness in others and the wholeness in life. The wholeness in you is the same as the wholeness in me." ❧

"We do no great things; we do only small things with great love."

– MOTHER THERESA

GRETCHEN:
SO MANY FRIENDS...SO MUCH TO BE THANKFUL FOR!

When I first met John Baker, I was struck by his caring. He was part of a group that came to Harmony Hill for a board meeting. When I first saw him, he was carrying a small bonsai plant. He was living on a houseboat at the time and the plant had somehow fallen into the water. He was so concerned about this precious bonsai that he hired a diver to go down and retrieve it. He brought it with him to the meeting to watch over its recovery. John, an attorney, was a tall man with a kind and compassionate demeanor. The next time he came out to a meeting at Harmony Hill I learned that he had just been diagnosed with mantle cell lymphoma. It was about that same time that we learned about the Commonweal program through Bill Moyers' "Healing and the Mind." John was often on my mind as we birthed our cancer retreat, and, in fact, he attended the very first one and even started the first support group with those alums.

John became a tremendous advocate for Harmony Hill, and I valued his wisdom as well as his friendship. It's okay to reveal it now: John was often the anonymous donor behind the challenge grants for a number of our fundraising campaigns. He was also willing to accompany me on my first meeting with Bill Gates, Sr.

As Harmony Hill reached its ten-year milestone, I knew we had to either fish or cut bait. We needed to grow to become sustainable, but there were enormous risks to achieving the growth that was needed. I wrote to Mr. Gates, who was as well-known throughout the Northwest for his civic leadership and philanthropy, as he was for his famous son and daughter-in-law, Bill and Melinda Gates. The Gates family was familiar in the Hood Canal area, for they, like the Nordstroms, had a vacation home just a short distance from Harmony Hill. I had met him before, but always in much more informal, social settings. Mr. Gates responded right away, saying he would be willing to talk with me as long as we didn't talk about money. I was fine with that, and set up an appointment. I was a bit nervous and asked John Baker to go with me.

As we ascended the elevator of Seattle's tallest building, I pulled some sprigs of lavender out of my pocket and inhaled it for the calm it provides.

"Put that away, Gretchen," John said, "You don't want to be holding that in front of your nose when the elevator door opens!"

He was right. Mr. Gates was waiting for us and led us to a large conference room with a dizzying view of the city and the Puget Sound.

Mr. Gates was extremely cordial. He asked John right away what his role was and John told him he was here as my friend, not as counsel. John proceeded to tell the story of his own cancer and how beneficial he had found Harmony Hill's cancer

> *"Everything I do, all of these blessings, everything I give, it all comes back to me ten-fold. I just give it away, everything I can... it's always a cycle. I give. It comes back to me. Then I energize it and put it right back out there.... It's the best blessing of all, to me."*
>
> – DOLLY PARTON
> (FROM *ON GRATITUDE*
> BY TODD AARON JENSEN)

program to be. Mr. Gates asked numerous questions about the Hill's programs and operations. While we were now ten years old, it was clear to him we were still a "start-up," especially since we had so radically changed our focus with the inception of our cancer programs. He asked if we had ever used the senior program called SCORE, through which retired business executives help start-up organizations. I told him that I had contacted SCORE but they told me they were not serving nonprofits. (Let me digress here to report that the very next day, the president of the Washington chapter of SCORE came out to Harmony Hill to see if he could help with anything. Yes, he had received a call from Mr. Gates!)

A comprehensive business plan was something Mr. Gates highly recommended. While we had a good sense of where we were going, we did not have a well-defined business plan at the time. At his suggestion, we hired a consultant to help us craft a true business plan. It took a full year to develop it. Mr. Gates had agreed to read it once it was written, so a year later I was back at his office, this time accompanied by Board member Mike Towey. Once again, Mr. Gates had a lot of excellent questions, the last of which was, "What do you need?" I reminded him that our original deal was that we were not to talk about money. He said, "Well, we're friends now, and I can see you're doing something that could be of value. Let me know by tomorrow what you think you might need."

It was a long night. We really didn't know what to ask for and we only had a few hours to put something together. The next day, with trepidation, I faxed to Mr. Gates a request for $75,000. It seemed like an enormous sum! The very next day I got a call from Mr. Gates and his words were ones we usually only dream of hearing: "Gretchen, you didn't ask for enough money!" He went on to explain that he had talked to Bill and Melinda and they agreed that our project had merit. "You need more money to get it off the ground. We're going to give you $200,000, which will break out to $85,000 the first year, $65,000 the second, and $50,000 in the final year. We want you to stay in touch with us, keep us posted on your progress." He concluded by saying, "Use this money for leverage to get other support, and don't come back."

We rejoiced in this amazing gift, arriving at just the time we could use it to move Harmony Hill to a new level of service and a new stage in its evolution. This grant, spanning 1998 to 2000, made it possible for us to bring on additional professional help to really get the cancer program up-and-running. ❧

The gift of giving

Gratitude generates the healing energy that emanates from the heart of Harmony Hill. Most people who receive that energy at Harmony Hill are inspired to stoke the spark of generosity in their own lives, to pass it on. The receiver of kindness and compassion then becomes the giver and in giving, is replenished. It is a perfect circle: endless ripples of gratitude, perpetual healing.

There are as many ways to give back as there are people whose lives intersect with Harmony Hill. Here's how a few of the alumni featured in this book have chosen to give back:

For **MAROLAN TILCOCK**, the act of giving back has rekindled her life.

"When I saw what Harmony Hill gave people – specifically what they gave to me – I wanted to give that to others. My experience there really showed me that something *big* was missing in my life. That 'something' was giving back, helping others, being generous; doing all the things we all *say* we want to do but never get around to doing.

"I think I was just like a lot of everyday people. The big change that happened because of my cancer and Harmony Hill was that I found the focus and the courage to do something good for the world, to give back. For me, it's about having that personal debt. I don't think everybody needs a debt to repay in order to give, but I think *I* needed one, to get off my butt and turn my life into what I really always wanted it to be."

Once she started on the path of giving back, Marolan has found the possibilities infinite. Here are a few opportunities for giving back that she's created:

Angels: "While I was going through my cancer, I started making these angels." Marolan's angels are lovely little beaded figures, slightly abstract, with tiny wings.

"First I made one for myself and hung it on my purse. I was at the Cancer Center when a woman in the waiting room was having a bad day. She'd gotten bad news and she was alone, so I was hugging her while she was crying. When I was getting ready to leave, I looked down at the angel hanging on my purse, and I handed it to her. I went home, made myself another one, and hung it on my purse. Then another person needed it, and I gave it away. It happened again and again and again. Pretty soon I was stuffing my purse with all these little angels and giving them away whenever I met someone who needed them. And now some of my little angels are hanging in the Harmony Hill gift shop."

Golf Fundraisers: When Marolan heard that Harmony Hill was trying to raise funds in order to match the Gates Foundation grant, she knew this was another opportunity for her to give back.

"I know many Microsoft administrators, so I introduced them to Harmony Hill; we organized a golf tournament and raised $55,000. And I'm going to keep introducing new administrators (there are so many at Microsoft!) to the Hill so the giving will keep growing and growing."

Cancer Support: "I've recently started working with people who have cancer. When a friend knows someone who's diagnosed, they'll often call and ask me for an angel. Then they started asking if I would meet and talk with that friend about my own experience, and I began meeting all these incredible people. Now I email some of them and give them encouragement. Or I make phone calls, maybe meet them for lunch. I don't give them advice, I just give them the sounding board of someone who's been there. I don't know that I would've had the courage to do that if I hadn't gone to Harmony Hill."

P2B: "During my search for ways to give back and thinking, in particular, about future generations, I founded a girls' group, **P2B** (which stands for **Power to Be**) when my daughter Hannah was in fourth grade. **P2B**'s goal was to connect elementary-school girls to the community, to help them do good — picking up trash, helping at the food bank. We wanted to teach the girls that they could make a difference – all they needed to help people were good ideas, some help from their families and a lot of hard work. Now the girls are in junior high, and I'm proud to say that they still value this group and all want to continue. By letting the girls come up with the ideas of who they wanted to help and how they could help, it's given them a stake in the success of each project. **P2B** has taught them how to run a meeting, how to communicate with care and respect, and about how giving pays them back, tenfold, in how they feel after helping others. We knew that having parents involved would make a difference, but we underestimated just how much an impact it would truly make. The events give the girls a special opportunity to work side-by-side with their parents, their friends, and their friends' parents. It's made communicating easier for all of us; it keeps those lines of communication open, while providing valuable time together. And it's created many memories filled with laughter and tenderness."

Marolan has also been part of the team of volunteers and staff who have been envisioning and planning support programs at Harmony Hill for children whose lives are affected by cancer in their families. Alums **PATRICK AND SARAH HEALY** are part of that effort, as well as **MICHELLE CLIFTON**, who also still plans to give back by opening a day retreat for women with breast cancer.

Whenever there's a Volunteer Day at Harmony Hill you'll find **CANDIE SCHMITT** and her husband **STEVE** there, along with a host of other alumni and friends of the Hill, giving back in hands-on fashion – gladly doing whatever needs doing.

The **FOBs** (**Friends of Barbara**) continue to give back – **ELAINE HOLLAND**, the marathon fundraiser; **MARJORIE LUCKEY**, the housemother volunteer. All the **FOBs** contribute time (like fundraising-committee volunteer **HELENA COHEN**), energy and money in support of the Hill. And **BARBARA RIEFLE**'s legacy is a giving testament.

There's a multitude of alumni who choose to give back by asking friends and family to donate to Harmony Hill – perhaps requesting those donations in lieu of birthday or Christmas gifts for themselves, as alum **HILARY GREENSTREET** does.

And alum **BARBARA OSWALD** gives back by offering an oasis of comfort and company in her B&B to individuals who are going through cancer treatment. Harmony Hill was the impetus for **JULIE BARRETT ZIEGLER** becoming a hospice volunteer. And **RICARDO GOMEZ** directed the proceeds from his book chronicling his cancer journey to Harmony Hill.

These are but a few examples of a few of the numerous people who perpetuate the cycle of gratitude at Harmony Hill, in their own lives, in the world. Every one of their stories is itself a gift, an open invitation to join the joyous circle. ❧

GRETCHEN:
SO MANY FRIENDS...SO MUCH TO BE GRATEFUL FOR!
... PART 2

Just as the first Gates grant was wrapping up, we received word from Kitty Nordstrom, shortly before her death, that she was willing to give us a longer term no-fee lease on the Harmony Hill land. She was offering us a 30-year lease, with two five-year renewal options. With assurance that Harmony Hill had a home at least through 2040, we could think seriously about growing our programs and expanding our campus. At that same time, we were informed that there might be funds available to us from the Seattle Foundation to make improvements to the campus. With this news, our board wanted me to go back to Mr. Gates and see if we could get further support from the Gates Foundation to help build the cancer program and expand our campus to serve more people. Although Mr. Gates had instructed us not to come back, given our change of circumstance I decided to invite him to Harmony Hill for a site visit. He spent a couple of hours with us and asked lots of questions. His final question was, "Gretchen, does the world need this?"

I took a deep breath and prayed I would find the right words to answer his question. I told him the story of one of our recent cancer retreat attendees who came to our door with an emesis basin because she had been vomiting frequently. She had a brain tumor and was living on Ensure because she was having tremendous difficulty eating. Even the smell of food made her nauseous. Harmony Hill purposefully prepares fragrant meals, so this last information posed an additional challenge for us. We gave her a back bedroom on the main floor of the main house. I promised her we would do our best to minimize the cooking smells, but also told her we could do much better than Ensure milkshakes. We hoped she would be able to join everyone at the dinner table. I described to Mr. Gates how, over the next five days, this woman was able to eat the food from our kitchen and drink nutritious smoothies we prepared. She and her husband were enormously relieved and amazed by the change in her energy and her outlook. We learned that within two weeks after attending the Harmony Hill retreat, she hosted a dinner party at her house for the alums who had been at the retreat and she even cooked part of the meal. She lived another six months, *and they were quality months*. She had time then to put her affairs in order and to say her goodbyes. "Mr. Gates," I concluded, "If you were that woman or her husband, it would mean the world.... So, yes, Harmony Hill is needed by the world – one person at a time."

Our second-round grant request was for $500,000, divided over five years. We submitted the proposal in early summer and we didn't hear a thing for months. This was unusual for the Bill and Melinda Gates Foundation, which was known for getting back to organizations within a few weeks. I asked Les Purce, from our advisory board, if he would advocate for us. Les did, but still there was no word. As we approached the end of the year we were uncertain how to budget for the coming year. Would there be additional funds to support our goals for growth?

Early in the new year I learned that John Baker, who had accompanied me on that first visit to Mr. Gates, was dying. John had had a stem cell transplant that was not successful. A few days before he died, John said to me, "Gretchen, do you have any requests for when I get to the other side?"

Almost immediately, I said, "John, please go find Elmer Nordstrom and ask him to somehow get word to Mr. Gates that we really need to have that grant funded!"

I stayed with John and his family for a few days and came home the morning following his death. Three days later, I was thinking about him as I walked down to the mailbox. I pulled out a letter from the Gates Foundation. Enclosed was a check for $150,000. The entire $500,000 grant was approved! I called John's wife, Gay, and told her that he was already hard at work on the other side. We laughed together and we cried. Such an extraordinary moment! ❖

The connections made at Harmony Hill aren't just to a place or to individuals. There is an alchemy that takes place here that is truly magical. The interconnectedness of all things is breathtakingly evident. A word spoken in caring and compassion can reverberate unendingly, touching lives and changing energies in people and places that have never heard of Harmony Hill. Gretchen has noted how Harmony Hill serves as a catalyst for a growing sense of purposefulness.

"When people take part in a Harmony Hill retreat, they aren't just helping themselves but others who are also at the retreat. When someone purchases a brick for our tribute path, they aren't just honoring a loved one, but are honoring the future of Harmony Hill and the many lives we have yet to touch. Even when a volunteer chops carrots in our kitchen or makes copies in the office, they are an essential part of bringing the healing beauty and power of the Hill to others." ❖

STEVEN PONTES:
A LEGACY OF CARING

Steven Pontes was introduced to Harmony Hill by his friend Amba Gale. When she learned that her dear friend, a successful businessman and single father from California, had been diagnosed with an advanced gastro-intestinal cancer, she connected him with Gretchen.

Gretchen was immediately struck by Steven's upbeat nature and his confident optimism, even in the face of a grave prognosis. He attended a Harmony Hill cancer retreat in June of 2006, and from that point on, until his death in February 2008, Steven became a passionate and committed champion of the Hill.

He maintained a Caring Bridge site to journal about his experiences and keep his many friends and loved ones apprised of his progress. About his experience at Harmony Hill, Steven wrote:

> The retreat was 100 times more than I expected or imagined. First, it was in an exquisite area of the Pacific Northwest - the Hood Canal on the Olympic Peninsula – in a city called Union. It was absolutely, breathtakingly beautiful. Second, the facilities could not have been more warm, welcoming, conscious and life-giving. Third, the food (YES, I AM EATING AGAIN!) was unbelievably delicious. Fourth, the program, the staff, and the overall commitment of Harmony Hill are nothing short of brilliant.

> The one thing I was so looking forward to was meeting other folks with cancer diagnoses. As it turned out, our group included those who were recently diagnosed, others who had just completed their treatments, others who were cured, and others who were diagnosed as terminal. To be amongst this group, share our thoughts and experiences with one another, laugh and cry, and generally explore what is next together was an incredibly valuable experience that just continues to resonate with me. Bottom line: the Harmony Hill Retreat Center and its cancer programs are one of the biggest gifts I have ever received in my life. THANK YOU, HARMONY HILL!

Gretchen recalls that when Steven attended his first retreat in June of 2006 he connected easily with all the participants: "That's the sort of person he was - you were immediately at ease in his presence."

There was a woman from Portland at the retreat, Jane, who was struggling with a lung cancer diagnosis. Steven became a support person for Jane and her husband, even traveling to Portland several times to visit her at home or in the hospital. Jane later recounted to Gretchen that Steven's willingness to listen to her fears, and to offer hope and encouragement, helped her to stay strong and positive.

"She told me that no matter what journey her cancer would take her on, Steven's inspiration and support had given her the skills and confidence to get through it."

Steven's belief in the magic of Harmony Hill extended to committing to a leading role in Harmony Hill's Major Gift Campaign Taskforce. Drawing from his entrepreneurial business skills, Steven introduced a whole new world of friends and advocates to Harmony Hill and its mission. His sincere and eloquent description of his experience at the Hill and the difference it was making in so many lives brought Harmony Hill to the attention of many who would never have known about it.

Steven, himself, committed to raising $250,000 toward the Major Gift Campaign's goal of $1.5 million. Even as his health became increasingly fragile, he regularly volunteered for speaking engagements where he shared stories of his experience at Harmony Hill and asked for support so others could have the same healing experience. Steven had raised a large percentage of the $250,000 by the time of his death in 2008; the remainder of the pledge was met through donations from his friends and family.

In honor of this visionary and inspiring leader, the largest room in the Elmer & Katharine Nordstrom Hall was named in his honor. The Steven M. Pontes Performance Hall is where most events at Harmony Hill take place. It's generally where each cancer retreat circle is opened, and where, on so many occasions, people experience the deep and rich connections with others that remind them of life's gifts. The light that floods that room is also Steven's light.

One of Steven's many friends, Jay Greenspan, shared this passage from the Jewish Kaddish (memorial service), noting that whenever he reads it, he hears Steven's voice:

> When I die, if you need to weep, cry for someone walking on the street beside you. And when you need me, put your arms around others and give them what you need to give me.
>
> You can love me most by letting hands touch hands and souls touch souls.
>
> You can love me most by sharing your simchas (blessings) and multiplying your mitzvot (good deeds).
>
> You can love me most by letting me live in your eyes and not in your mind. And when you say Kaddish (prayers) for me, remember what our Torah teaches:
>
> Love doesn't die, people do.
>
> So when all that's left of me is love,
> give me away.

At another point in his Caring Bridge journal, Steven shared with his friends this comment: "Now the other part of the 'sweetness' this journey has blessed my life with is the kindness that each of you has showered so generously on me each and every step of the way - you have no idea (in spite of my continuously reminding you) what a difference it makes. Your kind wishes, thoughtful and genuine gestures, vibrant words of encouragement along with all of your support have been and continue to be a major source of inspiration to cause me to make each and every day a new opportunity regardless of the nature of the circumstances in front of me. My life is richer than I could have ever imagined - because of you...Thank you!"

Steven Pontes touched so many lives in so many ways, and he continues to do so - through the expansion he helped fund, his tireless example, and his words that live on as inspiration to those facing a similar journey.

"Being in an environment where one can confront cancer, in all its forms – full on and in all of its stages – is a life-altering experience...if you are open to it. My life is fuller and richer, and I am more curious, willing, and practical about the finiteness of life – a finiteness that, if one is willing to embrace it, is full of opportunities and experiences." ❖

Harmony Hill's "housemoms"

The VOICE nurses are a very special group who originally came to Harmony Hill as volunteer housemothers for the retreats and later evolved into a support and teaching community. "Each of us came to the Hill for different reasons and somehow a deep connection was made," recalls Kathlene Tellgren, RN, CEN, HN-BC. At the same time, Gretchen was looking for a community of colleagues, other nurses who shared her vision of being a part of the transformation to a holistic healthcare culture, and providing support and healing to healthcare professionals.

"Gretchen called, and we came," says Linda Covert, RN.

Dianna Blom, RN, BSN, CCMHP, notes, "As housemoms, we're there for the retreat participants in every way possible. We watch for any health difficulties and make sure they have what they need. We want them to feel nurtured and pampered. If they need to talk, we're there to listen. We're on the sidelines and in the background unless they need us. We see our role as holding the space so they can experience whatever they need to experience for their own healing.

"We're also there to support the facilitators. They're holding all the individual energy and pain from everyone in the room. It's a big job. It's such a privilege to witness the courage and the transformation of attendees, and to be a part of the magic that happens. I've seen it time and time again: when you come from your truth, the right thing will happen."

One of Kathlene Tellgren's most unforgettable experiences as a housemom took place in 2003: "I was invited to be housemother for a retreat that had been customized for the Sisters of Hope, a support group for women of color living with cancer. They came to Harmony Hill already knowing one another, so from the outset, it felt much like a reunion. Before the retreat even started, when I was introduced to a couple of women as they were checking in, they gave me big bear-hugs. They were welcoming me as much as I was welcoming them. I told them that my job was to be in the background and to help with anything they might need through the three days. They would have none of that. 'Oh, no, honey! You're part of our group! You're one of us now!'

"As always, we opened the retreat in circle and shared our stories. I was going through a very low point in my nursing career at that time. I was exhausted physically, emotionally, and spiritually. I shared with them that I was questioning whether I could - or should - continue being a nurse.

"They responded as one: 'We need you to stay!' Each of them shared how her own cancer journey had been lightened by the words, or the touch, or the reassuring and caring presence of a nurse. 'You can't leave. We need you.' That was such a powerful message, and a profound healing for me.

"I had come there to hold them and, in fact, they held me. It was a transformational moment in my nursing career."

The experience inspired Kathlene to write a poem, which she sent to the Sisters of Hope participants along with her thanks for the gift they had given her, the gift of renewed meaning and appreciation for her life's work.

> Sisterhood is not confined to bloodline or race or creed.
> It is going beyond to a sacred, vast heartspace
> unknown by human mind and reason
> to a deep connection born of suffering and hope.
> Sisterhood is opening to the loving heart that sees all,
> accepts all with compassionate recognition,
> witnessing the beauty of women friends and soothing
> all the pieces that threaten to unravel.
> Sisterhood is recognizing that the most
> important treasures given from the soul are gifts
> to be cared for by the receptive, listening heart
> with understanding that needs no translation.
> And sisterhood is love, simply
> without conditions or demands open and giving
> from wisdom that nurtures
> the next steps of life's journey.

A year later, when the Sisters of Hope scheduled another retreat at Harmony Hill, they asked for Kathlene to again be their housemom. ❧

SISTERS OF HOPE

The Sisters of Hope Cancer Support Group is a Tacoma, Washington-based non-profit organization whose mission is to provide a safe, comforting environment for spiritual and emotional support for women of color diagnosed with cancer. Its founder and executive director is Betty Mewborn, a dynamic woman and community activist who is herself a 13-year cancer survivor. Betty describes Harmony Hill as "one of life's precious finds."

"Walking on Harmony Hill's land for the first time is like slipping through a window of love, into another rim. It's a beautiful rim filled with smiles and sparkles, love, energy and enthusiasm, with open arms for everyone."

Of her own cancer journey, Betty says, "No one is the same after cancer. Most of us never fully know the thrills and joys of life until our ability to experience them has been threatened by cancer. Facing fear is the hardest part, but once you've looked cancer in the eye, you'll see the hope that you can get through it."

Harmony Hill offered a customized retreat for the Sisters of Hope in early 2001.

"The Hill helped us to bring positive thoughts into our lives. The love, joy, happiness, tears, laughter, and peace we felt there will always be remembered. The energy around us was so strong we could feel angels. For some of us, that was the first retreat they had ever attended. To feel so nurtured, so cared for, was such a precious gift. Combine that caring with the heavenly food, beautiful scenery, the warm fireplace, candles, hot tea, and soft music, and you'll understand why it was hard to leave when the retreat was over!

"We came back the next year, and have had retreats at Harmony Hill several times more. Harmony Hill reminds us what matters, and it puts us in touch with our own healing capacity. There's nothing like it!"

Cheryl Garcia attended a Sisters of Hope cancer retreat at Harmony Hill in 2003. She attended in hopes of connecting with others who were dealing with breast cancer.

"The feeling of isolation I felt prior to the retreat was tremendous, because everyone I knew was healthy and I was seriously ill. My family tried to be supportive and understanding, but could not provide me with the emotional connection I needed."

Cheryl recalls the powerful experience of coming together in circle with her fellow participants: "That provided us with the opportunity to release feelings - fear, anger, sadness - without being fearful about how our families would take them. I felt a deep sense of release after sharing my inner thoughts and having them listened to without judgment.

"I developed a deeper sense of acceptance and inspiration from the survivors that I could win this fight. The most important thing I took away from the weekend was a feeling of not being alone. I had developed a support network that I could use when things were tough.

"With acceptance of my cancer, anger and fear do not rule my days. I am able to be a more positive person and live my life more fully today, rather than worrying about tomorrow." ❖

"And did you get what
You wanted from this life, even so?
I did.
And what did you want?
To call myself beloved, to feel myself beloved on the earth."

– RAYMOND CARVER,
LAST FRAGMENT

JENNA HELM:
BALANCING LESSONS

Jenna Helm is a caregiver by nature, which is one reason she passionately pursued a degree in Health Psychology at Bastyr University. She was eager to complete her degree and Art Therapy courses when she was waylaid by life with a lovely surprise – she was pregnant.

"I wasn't supposed to have kids, but my wonderful daughter Kara came along. I wanted to be home with her for her first three or four years then I planned to return to school and finish my education."

When Kara was a toddler, Jenna was ready to go back for her degree and to begin her career. That's when issues stemming from Jenna's husband's Asperger Syndrome (a form of autism) interrupted her plans.

"The daily pressure of intimate relationships really exacerbates Asperger's issues and over time, those issues take their toll on a marriage. Jim just couldn't handle my going back to school or work, and I felt such a need to."

When a friend who facilitated the Seattle *Artist's Way* workshops was leaving her position, she asked Jenna to take over teaching for her.

"I was very excited about the prospect, and was busy trying to figure out what to do for Jim, how we could best continue to raise Kara together, while gearing up to teach the workshops."

And that's when cancer derailed Jenna's plans.

"I'd felt exhausted; my energy was just going away. Something was off, you know? There was that little nudge, that something's-not-right feeling. I kept going from doctor to doctor, asking what's wrong and the doctors kept saying 'Nothing's wrong.' Then I got a lump, and they thought it was a cyst. They said, 'You don't have the family background for breast cancer, you meditate, do yoga, you're young, you eat green, you don't have the risk factors.'

"I hear this story from people in their 20s and 30s all the time – it goes to Stage 4 because we're so young that they don't act on it as quickly. The cyst went into my armpit and I went back to the doctor. I *knew* it was cancer at that point. My body was telling me, 'This is cancer, you need to go into the doctor and don't leave that office until you've had all the blood tests and scans to find it.' I'd had cysts before, but I had this chilling, panicky feeling that they *had* to cut this one out. When I told my doctor that, she said many of her patients feel the very same thing, their body telling them to reject this invader. That cold, chill feeling – never ignore that. You have to be really assertive with your doctor because it doesn't make any sense, and if you have to, keep going until you find a doctor who listens.

"It was three years ago when they really caught it, though it was very apparent six months before that; and a year or so before that, there was that vague feeling. A peace came over me when I knew. I had faith and still do that I will get through it. I cried, though, because I didn't want to go through what my dad did."

Jenna was fourteen and living with her family in Kenya at the time her father was diagnosed with brain cancer. The family had to move back to the States and Jenna's mother had to rebuild her life at the same time she was caring for her dying husband.

"When my dad was going through cancer, there weren't as many medications and ways to control pain. It was an awful, pain-filled experience for him. Some years later, my four-year-old nephew had a sarcoma that was mistreated as lymphoma. By the time they realized their mistake, they just had to send him home to die. He handled his illness and his dying with such grace. It's a life-changing thing, to witness death – it's a lot like birth. I'm not afraid of that part. Like life, it's how you go into it."

When Jenna was diagnosed, she was told she was "herceptin-positive" (Her2+ or Her2-Positive.) Herceptin is called "the homerun drug" of all cancer drugs.

"It's the drug that people have lived on since it came out; they're still here. There is, however, a small percentage of people who are herceptin-resistant...and that would be me."

The herceptin worked very well for a little while, then it didn't, and it's been a tough ride for Jenna since then. She's been off and on chemo and a variety of drugs, as she and her doctors have sought to "keep the soup just right" for the last three years. To keep her alive.

"Metastatic breast cancer is a chronic condition and it's also a deadly disease. There are so many pink ribbons out there now, and breast cancer is considered very curable by most people. The metastatic group, we're the 'quiet group' – the battle's not over yet. There are a number of us in this boat and the number is actually rising. It's nice that they have these new drugs that make it a chronic disease, but I don't think the psychological and emotional support for living that life [with chronic cancer] is there yet. When you have such an extreme diagnosis, it's a difficult road to navigate.

"I could be here two years or twenty, no one knows. I've watched very healthy people with the same metastatic condition turn very quickly and pass away quickly. They did everything 'right' then they got a flu or an infection and they were gone. So I don't have an illusion about that. This is considered a chronic illness but one that will be the thing that kills me – unless there is a cure that comes before it does. I'm not afraid of dying; I just want to live my life. I don't want to have so many drugs in my body that I can't be in my life. I don't want to just be a body with a pulse.

"There's a drug coming down the pipe that I've known about for a couple years; it's supposed to help overcome herceptin resistance. I knew someone in the same position as I, at the end of her line, who took It in the trials at Johns Hopkins. Her cancer just went away; the herceptin worked, finally. At the hospital, my pharmacist keeps saying, 'Hang in there, the cure is coming; it's just in the process for FDA approval. Hold on.'"

For Jenna, life is an adjustment, day by day, as she learns the cycle of whichever drug she's currently on, how it affects her body, her mind, her energy and spirit. Day to day, sometimes moment to moment, she never knows what her pain level will be, when a treatment or a spasm will "take her down." The cancer spread to her lymph nodes, her liver, her clavicle, her spine and her hips. Her doctors stopped counting the bony lesions.

"People think once you're off chemo, you're going to feel better. It takes a long time for your body to recover. Your body is permanently affected, and you may not rebound. I'm lucky to have my background, to understand how pain works, and what it does in your mind, your adrenal glands. Even though I understood, everything changed. My brain was not my brain anymore because the pain had taken over. Your chemistry changes and you're not the same person. Pain mimics depression; you're not running on the same juice anymore.

"I had all these tools beforehand that weren't accessible to me anymore. Like, I was a yoga girl...then the doctors are telling me, 'Don't move, you could break your back because of all these lesions, you could be paralyzed. So I froze up, and thought, 'Well, what do I do now?' Dealing with a body that's compromised and now functioning differently has sometimes been pretty hard. Finding a good medical hypnotherapist was extremely helpful in managing the pain.

"I also do a lot of work with my naturopath and my psycho-oncologist so I don't lose myself mentally through this. You can really get lost in being a cancer patient. Once you're in the depths of ten months of weekly chemotherapy, you begin to lose your Self in this weird space of 'Chemo Land' and that can become your only world. "

Jenna's inner strength, her joyful, upbeat personality and her playful sense of humor have helped her remain buoyant. But she couldn't do it alone, and she's learned how to seek out the right people and to ask for help. In the process, she's learned more about healing during her cancer journey than any degree could confer. As one doctor told her, 'Now you get your Master's degree and your doctorate degree in one shot."

"Harmony Hill is one of the few places where you can really do that, in person, with others. The experience at Harmony Hill was a first for me because I'm a caretaker and I don't have family around to help; it was the first time I really felt like I was in this space of being taken care of. But not in a 'mother-hen' way.

"I knew I was in a space where I could really feel honored for listening to my body. In yoga class if I can only lift my leg up this far, no one goes, 'What is she doing!' It was fabulous to have that for just three days where I felt like I could just be myself. I can be crying and no one is going to be freaked out; and then I can laugh with you about the absurdities, laugh and cry about it at the same time. I needed that.

"The retreat I went to was a breast cancer group, and it was especially helpful to be in that space where that was the specific topic. There are many factors in breast cancer – how aggressive it is, for one. People may think, 'Oh, I must be doing something right because my cancer's growing very slowly. And people who have metastatic cancer think they're doing something wrong. Sometimes, out of caring, people want to tell you if you ate this or did that, you'd get better. You don't get any of that at Harmony Hill. Nobody came up to me once and said, 'Have you tried this?' or "If you just ate better...' or 'If you were more spiritually aware....' That was such a relief at Harmony Hill. Nobody was going to judge you if you drank a coffee or ate a cheeseburger, there was no judgment about how you choose to live your life.

"There were only two or three other attendees who were metastatic. Sometimes people who don't have metastatic cancer feel like they can't complain, they only had one or two little tumors. Well, one lump or 20, your world has just shifted, your sense of security has gone away, and reality has now hit, and you will be humbled; and we're all going to experience the same ramifications from it.

"Harmony Hill is a place of such acceptance. I haven't found that in any other part of the cancer world. And I could feel that acceptance even before I got there – it's totally 'come as you are.' I watched my housemother at the end of one session just sit there. I had barely moved in yoga session, sat in meditation and my tears were just flowing. Everybody else had left; I looked over and saw her just sitting there watching me. Best way I can put it, she was really holding the space for me, just making sure I was okay, letting me know without saying a word that she was there for me. When I was done, she was done. What she did was the essence of my whole experience of Harmony Hill. And I do plan to go back and just be in that space. I tell everybody I know about Harmony Hill. I say: just go. Go."

At Harmony Hill Jenna ran into a woman whose story was nearly identical to her own; her husband also had Asperger Syndrome.

"Our experiences were exactly the same. Our husbands, because of their disorders, they think whatever they feel, other people should feel. So, for example, if it's snowing outdoors but he's not cold, he doesn't put a coat on the baby when he takes her outside. The discussion I had with that woman that night on the Hill was so helpful. She had left her husband, and she said that leaving actually made him a better father. You can't negotiate the needs of the house because you have to deal with the Asperger-disordered individual's needs.

Jim fell apart when Jenna's cancer surgery was coming up. They weren't sure what was going on, didn't yet have a diagnosis of Asperger Syndrome (which can be difficult to discern.)

"I have compassion for him; he shuts down and can't read what other people are feeling, like, Kara's fear or my exhaustion. Still, it's confusing and tiring to cope with, and at least I'm not under any illusion anymore about what he's capable of. I think about his issues more than the cancer. Unless the pain is great, the cancer can kind of be in the background. I'm always thinking, 'How can I course-correct what's going on for him, give him the tools to be able to take care of my daughter if I'm not here?' It's still very challenging, but I feel like from all the help and all the angles that we've gone at this, I've done all I can do. Now I'm asking myself, 'How can I have my life, still honor him and still honor life for me and for Kara?'

"Kara has grown up with this. She's a very self-sufficient child; she has such a 'can-do, we'll figure this out' attitude," Jenna says, glowing with pride. "It's remarkable to see the wisdom in a child, especially one who's grown up with this. When I'm in pain, she doesn't take it on but she's aware of it, and she can offer support but she doesn't over-offer either. She can come up, pat me on the back, and say, 'You're okay, aren't you, Mom?' There's not a fear in her, she'll just kind of look at me, and go, 'You're getting tired, aren't you?' And she adjusts and says, 'Okay, then, we're not going to be able to go out and do things right now.' She's learned how to be flexible and to cope.

"Children need to be acknowledged in this process. Their needs often get pushed to the side. You're just trying to survive and so it's very easy to forget that they're processing things, too. Harmony Hill is putting together a program specifically for kids with the LiveStrong SuperSibs funding; I'm so excited about that. I found a therapist for Kara and she makes the call when she needs to go and wants to talk; she's very articulate and able to speak up when she really needs to.

"It's hard to think she's grown up like this, hard on me when I'm thinking, 'She doesn't remember me taking her to the zoo or hiking; she doesn't remember me active, only remembers me ill.' But the therapist assures me she's doing great, and says to keep doing what I'm doing because it's working.

"I've been getting a support system in place for her. That's the biggest reason we moved over here to West Seattle, where most all our closest friends are just five, ten or fifteen minutes away. And they're ready to step in and help out with her whenever they're needed. And Kara's school has been stable and incredibly supportive. We are so blessed."

Jenna has to keep making adjustments, to sustain her energy so she can be rested and present for Kara when she gets home. She has to parse her time carefully, and make different choices these days – about people, not about stuff. Being here for her friends, her daughter and Jim.

"People are remarkable and challenging and lovely. That's the miracle of people. I see people being so crazy, the world and economics so unstable, and at the end of the day, you know, it sounds so cheesy but all that really matters is the love." ❧

GRETCHEN:
ANY PORT IN A STORM

While I was undergoing cancer treatment, I was encouraged by my friend, Vivienne Hull, of the Whidbey Institute, to join her and several other women on a trip to Iona, a tiny island off the west coast of Scotland. Vivienne promised it would be a healing journey.

I was ever-so tempted. However, I felt that I needed first to complete one major aspect of the chemo experience – I needed to get my port removed. The port was the piece of equipment that delivered the chemo infusions into my system. I knew that it makes infusions easier and safer, but I *hated* that port and spent a lot of time trying to come to peace with it. When it was put in, I assumed it would be no big deal. After all, I was a nurse, I understood this stuff. I was dumbfounded, though, when the reality of the experience overtook my rational brain. I hadn't realized what it was actually like – *that it was a catheter that went into my jugular vein.*

It didn't help a bit that the surgeon who put it in had no bedside manners whatsoever! I felt that this lack even showed up in the port placement. It felt awkward and intrusive. I could feel it every time I turned my head. That awful old saying, "stick it in your jugular," came to me more often than I would have liked. I couldn't wait to get it removed and deferred going to Iona for a year so that could happen.

I had the best surgeon I could find remove it, then did everything I could to get myself back in a more gentle relationship with my upper chest and neck where the port had resided for so many months. Even today, I am still aware of the indentation in my chest, a permanent reminder of the bodily invasion it represented.

The whole port experience was particularly humbling and has made me much more compassionate when I review our cancer retreat applications and read about someone who has a port or is having difficulty coming to terms with one. Oh, yes, I've been there!

When I was in nursing school, there were some procedures we learned by performing them on one another – such as injections, IVs and nasogastric tube insertion. It was always a difficult part of the clinical process (whether on the "giving" or "receiving" end), yet it was very valuable. My experience with the port reminded me a bit of that experience – only a hundred times more invasive! I am very grateful that I will never have to put one in someone. ❖

> "It is one of the most beautiful compensations of this life that no man can sincerely try to help another without helping himself."
>
> – RALPH WALDO EMERSON

SUSAN KEITH:
POWERFUL INTENTIONS

Susan Keith sums up her philosophy with one question: "If you can't make a positive contribution to the world, what is the meaning of your life?" She answers that question with her life, giving generously from her heart and her many, considerable talents. Harmony Hill would not be the same without the time, energy and know-how she has devoted to its creation and evolution.

Susan was raised in a family where charitable giving wasn't even considered.

"My father was a blue collar worker and his attitude was, 'I work hard for my money, why should I give it away?'"

An ambitious student, Susan graduated ahead of her class and she was determined to begin working right away in order to be independent. Her first job as a part time receptionist turned into a full time job within the same company, and she was there for the next 38 years. By the time she retired, she'd held fifteen different positions.

Her first boss and mentor, Bud Schwarz, was an accomplished businessman and dedicated philanthropist. He believed it was his responsibility to tithe and that every business had the obligation to give back to the community which provided its livelihood.

"Inspired by Bud, I began genuine, deep community service while I was in my 30s. I was a single mom, so there were some tough years to slog through, often while working two jobs, but when the time came that I'd 'cleared the decks' and I *could* volunteer, I eagerly did so."

Her first volunteer experience was working the crisis line - a four-hour shift every week for three years.

"I had a management position at the time, and I'd leave the job with the weight of the world on my shoulders. After my four-hour crisis line shift, I'd leave thinking, 'I have no real problems at all!' It was the greatest opportunity for perspective," Susan enthuses. "Bud taught me about philanthropy and he encouraged me. He gave me support and the time to leave work early to get to my crisis-line shift."

Susan began to serve on boards, and at times, she found herself serving on three boards at one time. Altogether, she has more than 40 years' worth of board experience, which has proven to be a great benefit to Harmony Hill.

She discovered Harmony Hill via her long-time friend Margo. Both of them were active in the Avalon group, a forum for women managers in the corporate realm. Founded by Susan and another friend, Judith Nilan, its focus is on managing more from the heart than the corporate rule book.

"It was our Avalon custom to go on an annual weekend retreat together. As Margo had come to work at Harmony Hill in March of 2000, she suggested that we do our retreat that August at the Hill. I'd never heard of the place before, so I decided to go up and see where Margo worked.

"When I pulled up, I opened the car door and put one foot on the ground, and I just went, *Whoa! this is healing ground.* I have rarely ever had that kind of visceral reaction; it was so strong. And I didn't even know what kind of work they did....

"So we held our Avalon retreat there, and I first met Gretchen when she came down for dinner with us the first night. The next day as we were preparing to leave, I told Gretchen, 'The next time you come to Tacoma, stop by and see me and we'll have a cup of tea.'"

Long story short, Gretchen did call and they had a cup of tea that lasted about two hours. By the end of their lengthy conversation, Susan was holding an application packet for board membership.

Less than six months after she joined the Harmony Hill Board in February of 2001, Susan was chairing the marketing committee. It was only a short time later that the Board's current president had to withdraw from the position.

"Gretchen called me and Lu Farber, asking if either of us would like to be president. I was in my final year of my employment, preparing to retire; I had a lot of things to wrap up. So Lu and I got together and decided we'd propose being a team – she'd be president the first year with me as vice president, and switch roles the next year. We both had strong business backgrounds, and Harmony Hill was a pretty loose organization in those days. So Lu and I did the tag team thing and got infrastructure pieces in place. After two years, I stepped down from the presidency, though I was still on the Board."

The first major gift campaign ever undertaken on the Hill was led by Susan.

"When we made the decision in 2004 to stop charging for cancer retreats, we knew we'd have to expand our operations to create a sustainable plan to generate funds. It was probably 2006 when we got into the finite conversations about what a major capital/gift campaign would take.

"We hadn't done much in the way of fundraising before. The conventional approach is: first, you need a committee of people who can write $100,000 checks and second, they can go out and get others to write $100,000 checks. Well, we were pretty darned excited if we got a $25 donation, and $50 or $100 was cause for celebration!

"Sitting with Gretchen one day, I said, 'I get what the experts are saying but I don't know anyone who can write a $100,000 check. What I do know is that if we can accept pledges, I know at least ten people who can pledge $10,000 over five years. We can either give up or do things the Harmony Hill way.'"

After much discussion, it was decided that Harmony Hill would attempt to raise enough funds to meet the Gates Foundation's $1.5 million matching challenge. The deadline was the end of 2008. Susan was asked to chair the major gift campaign committee.

"I said, okay, if that's what it takes to get this started, I'll be the interim chair of the campaign. On the committee were Steven Pontes, Larry Nakata, Pam Hanson, Hank Riefle, Jane Caron, Judith Nilan, Ann Lovejoy and her husband Bud, and pro bono support by Clark Townsend (a professional development expert). Ann and Bud got a video specialist, Christopher Davenport, to film a terrific promotional video of the Hill. We asked the committee members to be *responsible* for $100,000 each – not to write a check for it.

"During the campaign, Steven [Pontes] died and that was a huge blow, both a personal loss and also the loss of a devoted champion of that campaign. At a Harmony Hill workshop/fundraiser dedicated to Steven, Lynne Twist (author of *The Soul of Money*) was a featured speaker. She had known and worked with Steven in prior years on the Hunger Project. It was Lynne's book that changed my mind about chairing the task force; in fact, she changed my whole outlook on asking people for money for a cause.

"A few months after the workshop, Lynne spent two hours with us, talking about Steven. She suggested we ask Steven's friend Jay if he and other friends and family of Steven's would be responsible for Steven's part of the campaign. We reached Jay that day, and he agreed to get a whole group of Steven's friends and family to meet Steven's commitment.

"That really re-mustered our morale and we proceeded with the campaign. We knocked on every door we knew. We were determined not to leave that money sitting on the table; Steven would never forgive us!"

With a lot of last-minute prospects to close within just days of the deadline, $90,000 was still needed to meet the goal. A big snowstorm hit, so Susan and the committee members were stranded in their homes. Undeterred, they sent email blasts in a fervent push to the finish line.

"We made it!" Susan says, her eyes beaming at the recollection. "It was the most inspiring thing to have people pour their hearts out because Harmony Hill needed them.

"People understand the depth of the work that's done here and that it's *transformative* work. There aren't a lot of places on our planet where genuine transformations take place on a regular basis. To be able to transform people who are having a cancer experience is to give them their lives back. And it's magic – to them and the people around them."

"The capacity to hold powerful intentions and to implement the actions that support those intentions can move the world. We've seen that time and time again at Harmony Hill. *If you do not set limits on your horizon of possibilities, you'll be amazed to discover what can be accomplished.*" ❖

> **"**There are some things you learn best in calm, and some in storm."
>
> – WILLA CATHER

Hard-won wisdom
from Jenn Helm's journey

Undiminished by her own health issues, Jenna's passion for holistic wellness and healing motivates her to share her experiences and resources with others living with cancer.

"One of the most important things I would like to impress upon everyone is that **being open and in touch with your body and practicing meditation** are extremely helpful practices – preferably developed before you have any major stressors happen in your life, such as cancer or divorce. If you allow yourself to listen to your body and not be afraid, it's very helpful in navigating what you need to do. Even though I had that training, I let fear stop me for too long from really pursuing the validation of cancer. I didn't want that to be what was going on. When the doctors would say, no, it's not cancer, I wanted to believe them. I'd go, 'Okay, thanks! I didn't really want that anyway.'

"**Trust your connection with your body**, and if you do that, you're more likely to catch it early – if you're not afraid. I think a lot of people think they don't really want to know because they think they can't handle it. But they can. They just have to get over the fear of not being able to handle it.

"I read in a psych journal that 50% of healing comes from the placebo effect from the trust you have in your doctor. The first doctor I saw was a lifesaver. He had developed the breast MRI and was an internationally-respected person in this field. He had personally overcome two cancers that were supposed to be incurable. And there were signs posted all around his offices: *Trust your intuition. Listen to your body. You know what's going on; make your decisions based on that. You don't need a diagnosis from a machine.*

"He told me, 'Take your time. Do not treat this like an emergency. If you have anybody treating it like it's an emergency, remember you have every right to take your time to make choices. He was my angel. I was so blessed that I got to see him first. He gave me the groundwork; he told me to trust my background and my intuition."

When she went to a cancer center for a second opinion, Jenna was told in a very abrupt way that her cancer was going to her liver and then her bones and then she would die. And there was nothing they could do to help her.

"I think they gave me this girl right out of med school who had never dealt with this before. She was talking like she was reading a textbook to me. She didn't know any better. Whereas my doctor is an expert in her field and has seen everything so she knows not to go, 'This is what's going to happen,' because she knows this disease is not linear.

"So listen to yourself first then get other people's opinions. If you go to a lot of

> **"**Sometimes, our light goes out but is blown again into instant flame by an encounter with another human being. Each of us owes the deepest thanks to those who have rekindled this inner light."
>
> – THICH NHAT HANH

different people, you're going to hear a lot of different opinions. **If your doctor is not listening to you, change doctors!** So much more healing happens if you can trust and relax."

Create your own toolbox: Jenna created a lifeline for herself, one she calls her "toolbox" for when she's really in need.

"When I was in a good space, I wrote a whole list of friends I can call – who for what, places I can call, what exercises work for me on given days, books that are helpful at different points and why they're helpful. When you're really in the middle of it and you're tired and you can't think and you just don't know what to do for yourself, I look up at the 'toolbox' I've posted on the wall, and I have all this information plus affirmations from my hypnotherapist written on the other side of the list. So I wake up and the very first thing I see is a wall of support. And I'll go, 'Okay, I can't even think – what do I need right now? Oh, yes, a bath! A bath is something I really need when I'm in pain!' I know that sounds strange but when you're really in it for a long time – metastatic, chronic for years on end – you can really get too tired to think straight."

Daily inspiration: The best thing Jenna's found to do for herself each day is to read something spiritually-based, a very short something.

"Just three pages with an affirmation at the end," she says. "When I wake up and I do that, it helps me ground into who I am before I move and my body goes, 'Oooh, I don't want to move'...or go to treatment or whatever the day brings."

Support, support, support: Jenna also found it vitally important to find a good, emotionally healthy group of people who are going through the same experience.

"I'm in a wonderful group online called *Crazy, Sexy Cancer*. I was a little hesitant at first, but I finally went to their metastatic forum. I had checked out several other online support groups and found they were very fear-based. But the CSC group was so full of life! They were living with canes and walkers and being laid up in bed and they still had this – what my nephew had, this attitude of, 'Okay, this is just life, we're going to deal with it and we're going to get through it; and we may die but we're going to help each other come to peace with what we've got to come to peace with, and we're not going to just give up.' It has been invaluable. Finding the right group for you is important. There are some schools of thought, like, 'Don't talk about it, don't think about it and it'll go away.' I kind of went that way for a while, just hoping it would go away, but I found it more helpful to find a group where I can talk about it, openly and honestly.

"And Harmony Hill is one of the few places where you can really do that, in person, with others who know exactly what you're going through. A place where there's no judgments, no pity – just understanding, support and acceptance."

Finally, and above all, Jenna urges, **"Never, ever give up on yourself!"** ❖

VICTRINIA RIDGEWAY:
LIVING TO A HIGHER CALLING

Victrinia Ridgeway is a force to be reckoned with: passionate, compassionate, creative and vibrant. Hers is often the first voice potential participants hear when they call Harmony Hill, and she takes each call very seriously.

"It's important to me that they feel that they have someone who understands them, that they have a friend before they get here," she says. That understanding has been hard-won and deepened by Victrinia's own personal experience with cancer.

Her journey to the Hill begins with a blossoming love story. Victrinia and a fellow in Tulsa named Eric made a connection over the Internet *vis a vis* their mutual passion for the art of bonsai.

"I was looking for work, and he – 'Google Ninja' – was looking all around on the Internet, and he found this job and told me, 'That's not that far from where you live and it is totally up your alley.' He said, 'You *are* applying for this job!'"

She did apply and she did get the job. Though she's always done nonprofit, social-services types of work, Victrinia immediately discovered that Harmony Hill was like no other place she'd worked before.

"Harmony Hill is not of the world. Not of the world in any way shape or form. There are many things we do simply because it's the right thing to do – though maybe not the easiest, least expensive practice. It's living to a higher calling.

"Apart from Harmony Hill's mission, what is *unique* is how we function as an organization. We have a standard of being compassionate, mindful of each other's needs, being supportive of each other.

"When it's really hectic, with back-to-back retreats, I'll sometimes work a long day and my co-workers kind of rush in, yanking little irons out of the fire to get things to simmer down because they all care that much. The cool thing is that when things quiet down, I get the opportunity to do the same thing for others. That's what we do. And that allows us to create an experience that surpasses what you can get elsewhere."

"I couldn't have a more perfect job anywhere else. At Harmony Hill, we do what we're best at; my role's been in constant evolution."

Victrinia was hired as a part-time program assistant; next, she became the full-time cancer program assistant for one-day retreats and weekly yoga. As these programs got pumped up, in addition to her role as program assistant, she began doing some marketing, plus IT. She's also become the unofficial photographer, artfully capturing many beautiful and often magical moments on the Hill.

"Personality-wise, I'm both logical and emotive. The logical side of my brain gets all happy when I'm playing with computers, science, and situations that are all highly predictable. I'm a geek by proxy – my dad and my husband are both geeks. And then I'll sit down and read an applicant's story and just...cry. These two positions – program assistant and IT person – so diametrically opposed to each other, create this beautiful balance in my life that wouldn't happen anywhere else."

Victrinia had been at Harmony Hill for nearly two years when she acquired a new "role" as cancer survivor. At a one-day "Tools for the Journey" retreat, seated in the circle for the first time as a member of the cancer retreat herself, she revealed her diagnosis and treatment.

"When I made the announcement at the retreat, that's when it hit me that I wouldn't be able to have children. I was the poster child for early detection – didn't have to have chemo, radiation, just had to go in for three-month checkups after the surgery. It would have been easy for me to discount my experience because it wasn't as bad as others' in the circle. But I realized my experience is very valid. My cure came lightly, but it will always be a daily part of my life. I will have to face the loss every day."

"The most amazing thing was how it changed my work, what I do here. Most people who work here aren't cancer survivors. People are surprised. They think that we're all cancer survivors. It's like when I worked at Catholic Community Services, they thought we must all be nuns.

"My cancer changed the language of every conversation, the way that I could empathize, the depth I could connect with cancer retreat participants. Now suddenly I had a story I could share with them on the phone to let them know I understood, that I understand the depth of their fear and their suffering.

"I still regard the diagnosis and going through all that as a blessing. For one thing, my then-fiancé, Eric, was so amazing. If there had been any doubt in my mind that this was the love of my life before, that doubt was completely obliterated. His caring, compassion, his being there for me.... He made me laugh when I needed something to be joyful about. He said, 'I will buy you all the children you want, and I will pay someone else to potty-train them for you.' And I knew we would find a way together to make a family."

Eric and Victrinia were married in May 2009; their bond deepens and blossoms every day.

And at work, Victrinia gets love notes all the time from people who have attended Harmony Hill's cancer retreats.

"The satisfaction I get in my soul from this work – there's no gift to compare. I'm very grateful and humbled by it. When they're effusive in their thanks, I sometimes don't know what to do with it. It's not me, it's them. I do this because of what they bring out in me.

"After my cancer experience, I became the servant who served with my heart completely changed – everything became more precious, more treasured, in that sequence. *Given the choice not to have cancer and the changes it made in my life, I don't know that I'd give it up. It makes me who I am. I was being molded into this lifework.*"

And for Victrinia, the work never gets old.

"Every time I come down to the office from group, I always say, 'This was the *best* group *ever!*' Every time. And it is. Everyone brings something...each person, each group is unique.

"You just don't know, you never can quite tell the impact you're going to have on someone's life. I treat each one of them as if it is the most important relationship in the world. Because it could possibly be – for them and even for me, in the long run. It could be the most precious and sacred relationship and opportunity, and I just don't allow one of them to go by. Not one." ❖

"Let yourself be silently drawn by the pull of what you love."

– RUMI

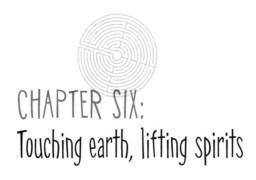

CHAPTER SIX:
Touching earth, lifting spirits

"It was a combination of the beauty and spirit of the place. We all felt deeply inspired by Gretchen's passion and vision for Harmony Hill and also sensed we were on a similar path. The values and consciousness present at Harmony Hill were important to us as the space we work in greatly supports the deep work we do with people." – GEOFF FITCH, PACIFIC INTEGRAL (ON WHY HIS COMPANY HOLDS MEETINGS AT HARMONY HILL)

Thousands of volunteer hours are devoted to maintaining Harmony Hill's spectacular gardens. In addition to an abundance of trees and flowers adorning the grounds, Harmony Hill grows many of the organic vegetables, fruits, and herbs used in the kitchen. Among the most dedicated volunteers is a cadre of women who are residents of Mission Creek, a Department of Corrections Center for Women in Belfair, Washington. Three or four days each week a crew of women from the prison may be seen weeding or planting the gardens, assisting with upkeep, and maintaining the beautiful grounds at the Hill. For many of these women, it is their first opportunity to work closely with the earth and to develop an appreciation for nature. Many acquire employable skills and, after serving their sentences, find work in the local communities and continue to volunteer at Harmony Hill. After their release, several women have brought their families to Harmony Hill to show them the work they did and introduce them to the spirit of the place that touched them so deeply. ❖

NEW BEGINNINGS:
THE LADIES OF MISSION CREEK

Constance worked on the grounds of Harmony Hill four or five hours a day, two days a week for about a year, while she was serving her sentence at Mission Creek. She remembers the first time she went to Harmony Hill.

"It was so peaceful there, so beautiful. And they were kind to us; they treated us like we were special."

She worked hard on the Hill. "We did so many things. I helped build the labyrinth; we planted, weeded, dug up all the dahlias; I helped transplant all the rose bushes – that was a big job! We built a greenhouse, wheel-barrowed dirt into the hillside for the Great Hall. And the fence. I helped build the cedar fence around the kitchen garden – I'm really proud of that fence."

The work Constance did at Harmony Hill made a difference, not just to the Hill, but to her, as well.

"It taught me how to get along with others and how to work as a group. I used to be a colder person, harder. I was all 'woe-is-me.' But I became more sensitive, more compassionate. It also gave me patience … and friends."

Since her release from Mission Creek, Constance tries to get out to Harmony Hill a few times a year to volunteer. Michele Raven has become a friend.

"Michele's knowledge of plants is incredible! She's an amazing person, and so is Gretchen. They are both so kind."

It felt good to be a part of Harmony Hill. Constance continues, "I know how important the work they do there is. And they do it for free – they are not-for-profit. I tell so many people about Harmony Hill. I have a niece with breast cancer; it's spread to her spine. I'm hoping she can attend a Harmony Hill retreat.

"It's such a special place. They knew where we were coming from, but it didn't matter to them. They were so appreciative that we were there, so appreciative of the work we did."

Another Mission Creek worker admitted that before coming to Harmony Hill she had never put her hands in the earth. She said that where she came from there had been no dirt – only a concrete jungle.

For Rita, memories of working at Harmony Hill were memories of "lots of laughter and lots of love." Rita was among the first Mission Creek women to work at Harmony Hill in the early '90s. She was incarcerated for a second time in 2007 and again worked at Harmony Hill.

"I didn't know what to expect at first. It was so different. In the early days, I came daily, Monday through Friday. Later, when there were more work crews, I came two or three times a week. We worked hard – nine hour days. Depending on the season, we'd be planting or uprooting and transplanting. We transformed the place to make it look good for the people who came out there. We also painted, built fences, poured cement – you name it. Once the whole work crew built a log bench together – that was fun. I learned how to use a chainsaw and other tools. Michele taught me how to build things. I still remember – that's going to come in handy someday.

"I also got to work in the kitchen. Sharon [Baker] would request my help. I loved cooking. I learned to make a buttermilk nettle soup – everyone loved it. And white chocolate mint cornmeal cookies – we were cooking healthy and the food was so good. Sometimes I would greet the guests at breakfast and bring them juice.

"We worked hard, but they spoiled us, too. They'd bring us fresh-brewed coffee, pies, cakes. There were often parties, and they never left us out. We were always included. They never looked at us like we were different for being incarcerated. They treated us with respect, like we deserved another chance. Gretchen was always so kind, so appreciative. She is a busy lady, but she always had time for us. She'd always stop and talk with us, and she always thanked us. And Michele was wonderful, too – I learned so much from her."

Most of all, Rita remembers the beauty of Harmony Hill. It changed her life.

"I'd never seen a place that was so beautiful, so peaceful. Even though we were working, it relaxed me. Being there made me reflect on my life. I took responsibility for what I'd done wrong and I knew that if another chance was given to me I wouldn't mess up again.

"The beauty of the gardens and all those flowers calmed me. Even today, when I see flowers, they remind me of the beauty and peace of Harmony Hill. I can carry that with me. Life is about choices. I saw that there. God makes everybody different and we can learn to get along despite our differences. I saw how life can truly be, how beautiful, how it can flourish.

"Harmony Hill is a good place for a person who is incarcerated. If someone is full of rage and not able to feel peace, they can go there and see that beauty, and feel a whole bunch of love. They get sucked into that loving energy – it's the energy of all the people who have been there. A negative person comes out positive."

Rita vividly remembers an amazing experience: "I had never seen an eagle before, but I dreamed about one. I dreamed it was circling around me. Then, the next time I went out to Harmony Hill, I was standing talking with Michele and another lady, and this eagle just flew down and soared around us. It circled us twice. It was huge, with wings so big. And it was so close I could see its golden eyes looking at us. Somebody told me later that was good luck."

She also remembers one time when Gretchen was away on a trip and the work crew decided to clear out her porch. It was piled with tools and equipment. They found new homes for all the tools and paraphernalia, and they scrubbed down the newly cleared porch.

"Then we built a prayer shrine and put candles all around it. When Gretchen came home and saw it, she was so happy! She loved that shrine."

Rita hasn't been to Harmony Hill for a while, but she plans to go soon.

"I'm going to bring my daughter and show her how pretty it is. And I'll show her all the work I did there. For me, going to Harmony Hill was a privilege and a blessing."

Michele Raven has worked at Harmony Hill for five years. As Facilities Superintendent, she oversees the grounds maintenance – it's a diverse position in which she may find herself troubleshooting a broken well-head in the middle of a frigid night, tending to a worker's injured hand, or designing the gardens and building fences. She has a lot of help, and among those helpers are the women of Mission Creek.

"Working with them is one of my favorite aspects of working at Harmony Hill," says Michele. "It's demanding, rewarding, and fun. Seeing these women come and go and hearing their stories can be heart-wrenching at times, yet the joy of seeing how this place affects them is profoundly heart-*warming*. They come here thirsty for beauty, and then, not only are they working amidst all this beauty, they're part of creating it. That, for some, is life-changing.

"The women from Mission Creek come here in search of healing, just as our retreat participants do. And for them to be able to contribute to the lives of strangers helps fill a deep void. It helps them rebuild some of what they have lost and start to envision another life for themselves."

Michele recalls one of many stories that have touched her to her core: "One morning as we walked up the hill – as we do every morning – I could see that one of the inmates was upset. She told me that it was the one-year anniversary of both her incarceration and her father's death from cancer. She was remembering how she and her mother were not able to get to the hospital to see him during his last hours, or to be with him when he died. The guilt and grief she carried overwhelmed her. When she finished her story, she stood still on the trail, sobbing, and she extended her trembling hands, desperate for some comfort. I held her. And so did Harmony Hill, as it holds so many of us while we take big or small steps toward healing, and as we begin accepting ourselves for who we are. Every day in this magical place, the journey continues.

"I have my own story of healing and magic related to Harmony Hill. Many years ago when I was a college student with no health insurance I faced some very serious health challenges. With no access to health care, I struggled on for ten years, until a baseball-sized tumor on my ovary and various other complications laid me pretty low. I was so fortunate to meet Linda, a wonderful Nurse Practitioner who worked at the health clinic in eastern Washington, where I was attending college. Linda became my ally. She took my case seriously, pulled some strings, made the right calls, and the result was life-saving surgery. I always wanted to thank her, but never got the chance.

"Fifteen years later, here at the Hill, one of our regular and wonderful volunteers, Mary Sunderland, brought her cousin Linda to Harmony Hill. She introduced us and we immediately recognized one another from all those years ago. I was flummoxed! And for Linda, seeing me in such a place and in a state of health and vigor conveyed my thanks more clearly than words ever could. Nevertheless, I did try to tell her how much her caring and efforts on my behalf had meant to me. You don't get a chance like that very often.

"But here at Harmony Hill, second chances happen all the time...." ❖

> "Our true home is in the present moment. To live in the present moment is a miracle. The miracle is not walk on water. The miracle is to walk on the green Earth in the present moment."
>
> – THICH NHAT HANH

GRETCHEN:
LABYRINTHS

Harmony Hill's first labyrinth evolved from the circle garden that emerged when I was rototilling during my mother's cancer crisis in the early '90s. In what has become one of the profound lessons of my life, I stopped hanging on as tightly as I usually did and allowed the rototiller to have its way. Instead of tightly controlled straight lines, the tiller moved in broad circles, changing direction when it hit a large rock or other impediment. The result was a beautiful garden that circled through a gorgeous variety of plants and flowers. People started coming to see it and to walk the circular path. Many commented on how peaceful and relaxing it was. At that time, I didn't even know about labyrinths, but someone described them to me and I suddenly knew that our circle garden was a labyrinth in the making.

Soon after I learned about labyrinths, I heard that the Reverend Dr. Lauren Artress, an Episcopal priest, whose book, *Walking a Sacred Path*, was the quintessential reference for those interested in labyrinths, was offering a class on labyrinth that very weekend in San Francisco. It was Tuesday; I called and they had just had a cancellation for the class, opening a spot for me. I spent an extraordinary weekend with an extraordinary woman, and returned home with the realization that I only needed to add a few turns and alterations to the existing path to truly convert the circle garden into a labyrinth. As soon as we made those changes, people started showing up. It was like they said in *Field of Dreams*: "If you build it, they will come." We didn't send out any announcements or do any publicity, but people seemed to know that the labyrinth was here, and they came to walk it. It was exciting and gratifying.

The problem was that as fall turned to winter, we needed to allow the garden to go dormant for the season, but people kept coming to walk the circular paths. It became evident that we needed a year-round labyrinth. The space that beckoned was an overgrown patch of land surrounding a Sequoia tree behind what we called the laundry house cabin. A group of kids helped me clear out all the blackberry bushes – no small task! We were left with a marvelous space that seemed made for a classic 11-circuit labyrinth – with the beautiful Redwood tree in the center. As Cindy and Gregg Shank were helping me roughly stake out the circles, each of us had the same experience: working toward the center, toward the tree, it felt like a magnet was pulling us. We could feel the energy radiating from the center; it was intensely powerful.

Eventually, this magical spot became Harmony Hill's shell labyrinth. The tree came to be called "She Who Knows," emblematic of her quiet wisdom and the strength she seems to impart. Unlike the garden labyrinth, the shell labyrinth can be walked all-year-round, but like the garden labyrinth, people just started showing up to walk it. They come daily and they are most welcome.

Harmony Hill became a participant in Lauren Artress' Labyrinth Project and we became one of the sites to which people flocked on New Year's Eve 1999 to usher in the new millennium. ❖

Sustainability is one of Harmony Hill's core values. Part of that concept is maintaining right relationship with the earth through recycling, organic gardening, use of nontoxic/recycled materials in housing, and careful, conscious consumption of resources. As the Hill has grown, this value has been at the forefront as decisions were made and expansions were undertaken. In 2006, the Elmer and Katharine Nordstrom Great Hall was completed. This spacious and comfortable building provides a welcoming space for meetings, retreats, celebrations, and quiet reflection. The Great Hall – a 2,000 square-foot room with a huge river rock fireplace and breathtaking views of the Hood Canal – is now where cancer retreats open in circle.

The Great Hall, like the Creekside Lodge was Built Green™. This certification means the structures were designed and built to be energy efficient, healthy, and to use sustainable resources. For people with severe allergies or compromised immune systems – a side-effect of many cancer treatments – buildings like this provide a welcome respite and an opportunity to experience restorative healing. ❖

BARBARA RAY:
CARRIED BY ANGELS

Harmony Hill draws together a broad collection of vibrant, creative, and bright people, people such as Barbara Ray. Barbara's life would make an interesting read and, happily, now in her spry 80s, she's writing her memoirs. An adventurous seeker with a keen sense of curiosity, she was attending a retreat at St. Andrew's when she first met Gretchen Schodde.

"It was late autumn in the mid-1980s; some of us were taking a stroll on the grounds. Walking towards us was this quiet, gentle soul. It was Gretchen. She meets everyone as if she's known them forever; she has this gift of sharing, inquiring, and being. And so, she told us a little about what she was doing there.

"The next year, I was leading the women's retreat at St. Andrew's with another member of St. Stephen's Episcopal Church. We invited Melissa West to lead the retreat and asked Gretchen to be part of the program, to tell us more about her plans for Harmony Hill. And so Melissa and Gretchen's friendship began."

At that time, of course, there was just the lodge, the yurt and the cottage, and the little old trailer that Gretchen lived in. There were leaky roofs and buckets in hallways; all the buildings needed a lot of work.

"I knew resources were scant in those early days, and as a lifelong networker, any time my friends were moving or downsizing, I would pile their stuff into my car and take it to the Hill. I loved going over there for the day and refreshing my soul in the simplicity of the place."

When she had out-of-town family visiting, Barbara would take them over to rest their spirits, as well. She introduced her nephew Jimmy to Harmony Hill, and persuaded him to consider making a grant from his foundation to the Hill each year for a few years.

Shortly after Jimmy's death, his sister and one of his board members, Ed, visited the Hill. The lodge was a bit chilly that day, and Gretchen apologized that the hot water heater had just failed. On the spot, without a moment's hesitation, Ed made an extra grant to cover the purchase of a replacement.

More than 30 years ago, quite some time before she discovered Harmony Hill, Barbara had her own experience with cancer. She was living far from home and family, dealing with breast cancer "at a time when there were no books or publicity, and – because cancer was treated as a secret – at a time when there were few people to talk and cry with."

Once she was officially a cancer *survivor*, Barbara volunteered for the relatively new "Reach to Recovery" program, to offer breast cancer patients and their families the understanding and support that she well knew was needed. The program was founded by a woman named Terese Lasser, who, after her own operation for breast cancer, persuaded the medical community that patients could benefit from the opportunity to talk with someone who had been through a similar experience. Barbara shared her experience and listened; she gave others the chance to ask questions and to talk about their fears and concerns, in order for them to make well-informed decisions about their health and their future.

A few years ago, when her niece Wendy (one of the next generation of her family in England), newly-diagnosed with cancer, was visiting Seattle, Barbara took her to Harmony Hill for a one-day retreat.

"She absolutely needed it," says Barbara. "And it was very meaningful for both of us to share the experience."

Gretchen has long been a part of Barbara's life; in 2006, during a day's outing together, Gretchen mentioned that she was soon leaving for Iona, Scotland. She suggested that Barbara join the group expedition.

"I hadn't been to Iona since my husband and I were there in the '90s; it was a magical visit. This would be the first time I would travel with strangers. Well, of course, I went. Two of the women in our group had wonderful singing voices and in the evening, after dinner, when we had finished a day of being cradled in that holy place, they would sometimes sing to each other. Throughout our time there, we were often drawn by the sound of their ethereal music, and would sometimes find them in one of the little chapels near the Priory, lit only by candles, and playing a Welsh harp or a penny whistle. One day we took a boat trip to Staffa Island, where they sang to the echoes in Fingal's Cave. The music of *Fingal's Cave* of Mendelssohn's *Scottish Overture* couldn't come close to the beauty of those voices and the lapping of the waves of the sea that day!"

"Iona has become part of the Harmony Hill experience. Gretchen has had the great foresight to take some of the nurses' groups there. It's all part of the kind of deep healing that takes place at the Hill on many levels. Gretchen is a guide; she brings all these people together and they become part of a quilt. She empowers, enables and participates in the creation that takes place."

Barbara feels "totally connected" to Harmony Hill and that Gretchen has long been part of her life.

"I look at Gretchen and marvel at how she renews herself and those around her, growing the dream exponentially.

"I know that I have been carried by angels, even though I've been a heavy burden sometimes! I recognize some of these same buoyant spirits around Gretchen and am aware of the immense privileges we are given." ❖

GRETCHEN:
HEALING STONES

A year later, when Vivienne asked again, I was eager to join her on Iona. I encouraged my 83-year-old mom to join us; Dad had died the year before, and I knew this adventure would be good for her, as well. She later reported that it was one of the best experiences of her life! I completely agree. Iona has become my sacred space of deep immersion in soul and renewal. As I write this, I have now been to Iona seven times – it has become a part of my life rhythms and is a treasured experience, place and people.

Iona is considered a "thin place," meaning the distance between the seen world and the unseen world is slender. Many call it a magical isle, and from ancient times it has been perceived as a place of healing. Only about one-and-a-half miles wide by three miles long, Iona is a place of beauty and mystery, a place where one's spirit can dance on the breezes and one's body can grow strong while walking its paths or combing its beaches. The rocks on Iona are said to be more than 2.5 billion years old, and there is a special rock – white with veins of green – that is found on one certain

> *"Everyone needs beauty as well as bread, places to play and pray, where nature may heal and give strength to body and soul alike."*
>
> – JOHN MUIR

beach and said to have healing properties. That first trip to Iona I found many "greenstones," as they are called, and brought them back to Harmony Hill. I have since been back to Iona many times – co-facilitating a retreat on healing and the soul with Vivienne Hull and Kathlene Tellgren. Each time, I "harvest" more greenstones to bring back to Harmony Hill and give to cancer retreat participants.

The largest greenstone I have brought back is one Kathlene found that is shaped like a large human heart. It's about 4x6 inches and must weigh seven or eight pounds. The whole top is a layer of beautiful green. The biggest challenge, of course, is carrying them back. When a customs agent lifts my bag and asks facetiously, "What do you have in here – rocks?" I just nod. I have also been fortunate that everyone joining us in Iona has been willing to take a few rocks back for me to give away to cancer retreat participants.

The stones I give are mostly quite small and are often put in people's pockets as a small reminder of their healing journey. Several participants have had necklaces or other jewelry made of them. Many people tell me they take them along as a talisman when they have a clinical treatment or procedure. I do the same. One time I completely forgot the smooth, beautiful greenstone in my pocket when I was having a PET scan. The x-ray team quickly spotted it, though, and asked me, *"What is that?"* I was embarrassed, but they just laughed. I suspect they see this with some frequency.

We have three stones from Iona that we use now as "talking stones" in our circles, rather than talking sticks. Two are greenstones, one shaped like a smooth potato with a beautiful heart outlined in green on one side, another in the shape of a small heart; the third is a large black and grey heart-shaped stone that is said to be 2.8 billion years old. It is wonderful to feel them become warm as they are passed around the circle from one person to the next, and to think of the collective energy that has held them from hand to hand and retreat to retreat. ❧

MARGO FLESHMAN:
FAITH IN ACTION

Margo Fleshman became friends with Gretchen Schodde in 1990 during a group excursion with the Rev. Carol Ludden to Cuernavaca, Mexico. After their return from Mexico, Margo and Gretchen stayed in touch. At the time, Margo was Executive Director for the nonprofit Washington Women's Employment and Education, and Gretchen would visit her office from time to time.

"She'd stop by my office with a bunch of flowers – always tucked into a cut-off plastic bottle – and we would talk about the trials and tribulations of working in non-profit organizations. Although I had seen Harmony Hill when I was attending a workshop next door at St. Andrew's house, I'd never spent any time there. A year or two after our Mexico trip, I was at a vocational crossroads and totally stressed out. I called Gretchen and asked her if I could go out to Harmony Hill and volunteer for a while. For two weeks, I worked in the gardens alongside the women from the prison; I also helped in the kitchen and with preparation for group visits. I spent so much time in the garden picking basil that Gretchen gave me the name 'The Basil Queen.' It was a time of total renewal for me."

In 1997 Margo changed jobs and became the executive director of Exodus Housing in Sumner. Around that time, Gretchen visited Margo and suggested that she begin working at Harmony Hill.

"I can't believe I actually switched, but in 1999 I went to work at Harmony Hill as Business Manager, even though I had no previous training in that position. I have no idea how Gretchen found the funds to hire *anybody* at that time. But she did, and I began a nine-year love affair with the Hill that continues to this day.

"To say there were lean times is an understatement. When I first started working there we had a very small staff and usually we would meet around the tiny kitchen table for lunch. One of our perks was eating leftovers. Sometimes there was an abundance; at other times, not so much. In the lean times, Gretchen would make her famous 'Gibson soup' [named after a brand of refrigerator]. We never knew what would be in it and, believe me, she put *everything* she could find in that soup!

"Luckily, it was also a period of tremendous growth, as well as an exercise in faith, at Harmony Hill. After a while, we were able to hire a qualified bookkeeper and I began to do more development of infrastructure. Eventually my position became that of Deputy Director."

In November 2008, Margo retired, but she hasn't lost contact with Gretchen, the staff, or the place.

"My experience at Harmony Hill gave me a whole new spiritual dimension. I now understand the difference between curing and healing; I saw scores of people healed by the experience of being on the Hill. I now believe in miracles.

"Over the years I truly saw faith in action. Gretchen has this amazing faith, and I saw it manifested time and time again. Her vision for the Hill used to confuse me and, at times, even annoy me. Now it amazes me. She held that vision. The word 'incredible' is probably used too often, but not when it describes Gretchen." ❖

❝ Every blade of grass has its angel that bends over it and whispers, 'Grow, grow.'"

– THE TALMUD

HILKE FABER:
A LIFE-LONG ACTIVIST

Hilke Faber gets things done. With a background in nursing, Hilke's life work has always been associated with being a strong advocate for person-centered health care, whether working as a nurse, a long-term-care ombudsman, a Health Representative for AARP, serving on various boards of directors (including Harmony Hill's), or volunteering in her current role as the Founder/Advocacy Coordinator of the Resident Councils of Washington. And she continues to be a strong advocate for nursing and the contributions that nurses can make to health care.

"Nurses have been underutilized. I see the opportunities that we have with the health care reform bill and the opportunities for nurses to deliver the much-needed primary care in our nation," she says. "Nurses are excellent providers for primary health care, able to take care of the basic health needs of most people."

Hilke and Gretchen Schodde met when she was with the Washington-Alaska Regional Medical Program (W/ARMP) n the early 1970s. The rural community of Darrington, Washington, had been unsuccessfully seeking a community physician for a long time, and their clinic sat empty. The nearest hospital, in Arlington, was a thirty-mile drive on a long, curving, treacherous road. W/ARMP recruited two public health nurses, Gretchen and Lynne Vigessa, for a pilot project to become family nurse practitioners providing primary care in close collaboration with physicians from Arlington.

"We made a health assessment of the community – baby delivery, CPR, acute ER care, pediatrics, etc. We then looked at the skills the nurses had already and what skills they needed to build on to deliver the primary care needed in Darrington. W/ARMP, in collaboration with the UW Schools of Nursing and Medicine, set up an intensive nine-week training, and followed up with preceptorships. The nurses spent time with an OB-Gyn physician, with Medic One and the ER at Harborview, with pediatricians, and so forth, in order to set up the community care clinic in Darrington.

"It was a 24/7 job. This rural health clinic and other W/ARMP sponsored demonstration projects for under-served communities were instrumental in working with the Washington State Nurses Association to get legislation passed that significantly expanded the practice of nursing."

After the Darrington project, Gretchen was recruited by the UW to get her master's degree in nursing. She then joined the Nurse Practitioner Program as an Assistant Professor for seven years, assisting in the establishment of many rural clinics and preceptorships for graduate nursing students.

Years later, when Hilke and Gretchen reconnected, Gretchen talked about her vision of what was to become Harmony Hill, about what she had begun and what she wanted to do in the future.

"Her vision is what sold me, and that is how I got roped onto the Board!" Hilke says with a laugh. "As I share many of the same goals that Gretchen expressed, I became excited about her vision, and offered my support of making this dream come true.

"I was on the Board at Harmony Hill for five or six years. We were always looking for money, barely surviving, with Gretchen living year 'round in a beat-up little trailer. When Carolyn Olsen's term as Board President was up, I co-chaired the board for two years with Mike Towey."

Hilke also helped the FIEs, as they were forging their union, to become better connected with the Aging Network and resources in Kitsap County. Theirs was a "beautiful model," that Hilke wanted to help succeed.

"Making a vision a reality is not easy. My key role, my strength, is connecting people, making connections in order to make things happen. That's what Gretchen does, too. Look at who all she's brought together to make her vision happen.

> **"We can complain because rose bushes have thorns, or rejoice because thorn bushes have roses."**
>
> – ABRAHAM LINCOLN

"I still participate at Harmony Hill – on the advisory board, at the Visioning, on the fundraising committees, and most recently, with the Nightingale Initiative for Global Health. I always help with the parking directions at SummerFest." Hilke laughs and adds, "Everyone kids me that it's the one time I can officially tell people where to go!

"I love being on the Hill. The minute you drive up, you feel instantly at peace. I start letting go as I drive onto the property, knowing that I'm accepted there for whatever, whoever I am. There's a tolerance there for everybody. It's such a healing place. The food is healing, the gardens, the labyrinths; the whole environment is conducive to healing. Even in the early days, in its rugged state, it was still healing. That's unique to anywhere else I've ever been." ❧

BUD ALGER AND ANN LOVEJOY:
LIVING ABUNDANTLY

For four of the six years they were married, Bud Alger and Ann Lovejoy dealt with the daily realities of cancer. Prostate cancer, once in long remission, now emerged front-and-center in their lives. Bud was living in constant pain.

Friends told them about Harmony Hill and suggested they participate in a three-day cancer retreat. They were assigned a date in August 2007, but received a call in

January of that year telling them a spot had opened up that very week and asking if they could come. With a little effort, they rearranged plans and arrived at Harmony Hill on a wintry Friday afternoon. "We were so incredibly glad we did," recalls Ann, Northwest garden expert and author.

"For me, being with so many others who really knew exactly what we were going through was amazingly healing. If I wanted to cry, there wasn't somebody asking me if I was okay. Of course I wasn't okay. But at Harmony Hill, it's perfectly okay to not be okay. Everybody understands. Everybody speaks the same language. It gave us a peer group and a core of people who understood everything we needed to say without a lot of explanation."

While among other people fluent in the language of living with cancer, Ann and Bud had numerous "aha" experiences. Paramount among them was the realization that "we were both holding back to protect the other. We saw how we could open up in complete honesty – that realization made everything simpler and less stressful for both of us. The wonder of it was that the openness continued. For weeks afterward, more of what we learned kept appearing in our daily lives – the experience of Harmony Hill just goes on and on.

"Like so many others," Ann continues, "Bud and I found that cancer brings many gifts in its wake. Bud was always quick to say, however, 'Cancer is a gift, but the wrapping sucks.'

"We were in a community of grief and a community of hope. Both of those emotions come in and out of our lives, washing like waves at any given time."

Gretchen recalls meeting Bud and Ann when they came to a Harmony Hill cancer retreat early in 2007: "Bud was very frail; he was short of breath after any exertion. I think they both thought he was dying. Because of his frail condition, we were watching him closely. And over the course of those few days, we saw something shift in him. He became stronger, more vital. We watched his life-force return and expand as he connected with other participants and with his own capacity for healing. Both of them told me they no longer felt he was dying from cancer – he was living with cancer ... and the emphasis was on *living*."

Ann marvels at the courage, the humor, and the dignity with which Bud faced his illness, and his appreciation for just being alive.

"He woke up happy, just because he did wake up. It was inspiring to live with someone who embodied such delicious pleasure in life.

"In his final few years, Bud was able to realize his deep desire to live a life of service. He took the skills and lessons gained at Harmony Hill on the road – speaking to groups about the possibilities the Hill offers to individuals and family members dealing with a cancer diagnosis. He also started a support group for men facing serious illness and disability." It has continued even after Bud's death in fall 2010.

Both Ann and Bud joined the Harmony Hill Board and became active members of the Major Gift Campaign Task Force. Bud was instrumental in the production of an informational video that was developed during the Gates Challenge Grant fundraising effort. It's a powerful testament to the transformational power of the Hill experience.

The video can be seen on Harmony Hill's website. It features Ann, Bud, and many other individuals whose stories are told in this book.

Ann has taught a number of classes at Harmony Hill. She wrote articles about the Hill and edited the latest version of the cookbook. Her advice, consultation, and work in the gardens of Harmony Hill helped transform them from beautiful to breathtaking. She also secured donations of thousands of dollars' worth of perennials, and helped the Hill fulfill its commitment to sustainability and organic practices.

Over the course of four years, Bud and Ann became vigorous ambassadors for Harmony Hill, spreading the word at every opportunity. Their message was simple:

"Harmony Hill is such a healing place …its very atmosphere promotes healing. We came to Harmony Hill focused on dying and left with a new focus on living with cancer. What a difference!" ❖

"In the end, there is really nothing more important than taking care of the earth and letting it take care of you."

– CHARLES SCOTT

ERIC BLEGEN:
CHANGING THE WORLD

The state of Washington is a long way from Wisconsin, where Eric Blegen grew up. He moved to Olympia in the '80s to attend Evergreen College, majoring in political science and German. In 1993, he was still living in Olympia and playing in a musical band, and he and his band mates were seeking a house large enough and reasonably-priced enough to share. When he found one in the tiny town of Union on the Hood Canal, Eric immediately felt, *"This is where I have to be."*

The house was owned by Andy Bell (who was well-acquainted with Gretchen Schodde and had served as President of the Harmony Hill Board). Over the course of what became and continues to be a sound friendship, Andy told Eric a little bit about Harmony House, as it was then called, and one of Eric's house/band mates worked for a while in the kitchen. For several years, that was the extent of Eric's knowledge of Harmony Hill.

When Eric met his future spouse, Matthew, in 1998, he moved to Portland, where they opened a restaurant in the city. But Eric kept the house on the Hood Canal. When Eric and Matthew left Portland, they headed for Union and made that house their home. That's when Eric applied for a job at Harmony Hill.

"I had known about the Hill for seven years when I saw an ad in the newspaper: they were looking for an executive assistant. I really needed a job and was excited that I might have a chance to work right in Union and at a 'cool' place. All I knew was that it was an organization with a conscience and that it had great gardens."

He applied for the position and was scheduled for an interview on September 12th. He and Matthew then made time to spend a peaceful week together in the Olympic Wilderness, far removed from people, phones, and newspapers. They walked out of the wilderness on September 11, 2001. Eric had his interview at Harmony Hill the next day.

"It was a strange and rather surreal reentry to the world and to the beginning of a new role for me.

"I'd had some previous office experience in administration, bookkeeping, and management. So I was hired; I started as Gretchen's assistant, then I took on bookkeeping and capital project budgeting. From there, I began writing small capital grants, then assumed responsibility for capital project management and planning, then supervision of facilities employees, and finally became Deputy Director.

"One of my proudest accomplishments was having taken the lead role in writing and budget creation for the Gates Foundation challenge grant in 2005. I have also been the lead planner and manager of all of our major construction projects since 2004 (the Creekside, Great Hall, and Gatehouse buildings), as well as many infrastructure projects."

Over the past decade with Harmony Hill, Eric feels that he's grown a great deal, both personally and professionally.

"Harmony Hill has given me room to explore new areas and develop new skills. You learn a lot about yourself from managing others – that's something I hadn't expected. You have to know your own issues, strengths and weaknesses in order to help others develop their best abilities.

"My work at Harmony Hill has exposed me to a whole community of people I would not have otherwise known. And it's given me the opportunity to have an important, positive impact on the lives of program participants."

Eric considers his impact to be "indirect," in that his job doesn't usually involve directly interacting with people who attend the retreats. But there is one family to whom Eric – quite directly – made a great deal of difference.

"Over five years ago, our friend Tom was diagnosed with colon cancer. Matthew and I had met Tom and his wife Marie through their daughter Sara, who was a friend of Matthew's from graduate school. It was at Sara's wedding that we were introduced and struck up a surprisingly strong friendship with Tom and Marie.

"Sara and I began trying to figure out a way to get her dad to come to Harmony Hill for a cancer retreat. Marie was very receptive to the idea, but Tom wasn't. A pragmatic engineer, Tom had a stoic attitude and a staunch 'nuts-and-bolts' view of the world – just the kind of man who often thinks a place like Harmony Hill 'isn't for me.' Some men seem to dismiss programs at Harmony Hill because they think it's too feminine a place, too 'woo-woo.' It can be a challenge to convince them to give it a try.

"Marie had expressed that she and Tom were having difficulty communicating and dealing with emotions brought up for both of them; Tom's resistance to processing his own emotions or to validating Marie's was straining the relationship. Over the course of the year after the wedding, we all continued to work on Tom, and eventually he agreed to attend a retreat with Marie. This was a big accomplishment, and I admired Tom for his willingness to step outside his comfort zone."

Sara dropped her parents off at Harmony Hill on a Friday and spent the rest of the weekend at Eric and Matthew's home. On Sunday, the end of the retreat, Sara picked up Marie and Tom and drove them to Matthew and Eric's for dinner that evening.

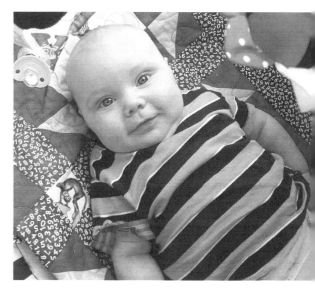

Eric and Matthew's son, Gus, born in April, 2011.

"It was instantly plain to us that it had been a profound and very positive experience for both Tom and Marie. They looked relaxed and were very affectionate with each other, very easy. They had made some real connections with the other couples in the retreat. Tom had bonded with two other men, in particular – men who were also professionals and who, like Tom, had an equally low 'woo-woo' tolerance. All of them had gotten past their preconceptions and found their world views were changed – for the better.

"It was deeply satisfying to me to know that this change had happened because I referred Tom and Marie to Harmony Hill. Over the course of the next year, Tom did well and returned for SummerFest the following year and actively participated in the Circle in the Great Hall that year.

"Tom died about six months ago, and his family is, of course, grieving. But they had over two years together after their Harmony Hill experience, and during that time, they used the tools given them at the cancer retreat. Their lives were fuller, more loving, and more connected with one another's because of that. This is the kind of experience that takes place all the time at Harmony Hill, and knowing that I help make those retreats happen is deeply satisfying.

"*Our mission is to transform lives – not to make widgets or a profit – to change lives, and to thereby change the world we live in for the better.*" ❖

❝ What is life? It is the flash of a firefly in the night. It is the breath of a buffalo in the wintertime. It is the little shadow which runs across the grass and loses itself in the Sunset."

– CROWFOOT, A LEADER OF THE BLACKFOOT NATION

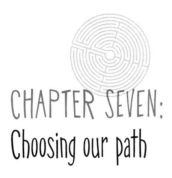

CHAPTER SEVEN:
Choosing our path

"If I didn't have cancer, would I have more energy? Would I have done more or be doing more? I don't think so – I think I would be doing less. 'I'm only 29,' I can imagine myself thinking, 'I have time.' And I do have time – enough time to do whatever there is time to do in the time I have. I know, however, that there are things I don't have time to do. I don't have time to go meandering unconsciously through my days. I don't have time to wake up next year and discover that I would have done it differently. I don't have time to follow-up on should-do's or have-to's. I'm too busy filling the days I have fought for with get-to's and want-to's; too busy making a life out of the endless possibility that lives inside each moment." – ROSE HILL, 2005

For many people whose lives have been touched by Harmony Hill, the gift of the Hill is the connection or re-connection to their life's path.

In many ways and for many people, cancer is a teacher and a guide. The experience of cancer – whether one's own or as witness to another's – often awakens us to our path and sense of purpose. Of course, cancer isn't the only means to such an awakening – but it is one that certainly gets our attention!

Our lives are so crowded with complexities, so bombarded by noise, so distracted by the hustle and bustle around us, that it's easy to lose our way. Instead of walking a labyrinth that always leads us to center, it feels more like we are walking a maze that continually offers wrong turns and dead-ends.

Being put in a position where we have to stop, where suddenly the familiar is gone – replaced by the topsy-turvy and the surreal, and where we have to face fears that had been crowded out of our lives – invites us to re-examine and re-evaluate, to look at where we are and ask if this is where we want to be.

When life comes down to the most basic questions, it becomes natural to answer from our most authentic self. The choice isn't "to be or not to be?" it's "how shall I be?" and "what's really important to me?"

A natural extension of asking – and answering – these questions for ourselves is to direct more and more of our energy toward those things that make our hearts sing, and away from the people and activities that drain us and deplete us.

Whether the connection to our life's path is made as a result of a cancer diagnosis, a loved one's struggle with illness, the inspiration of a stranger's story, or an awakening by other means – gentle or harsh – following our true path is the greatest gift we can give ourselves ... or the world. ❖

"The heart of most spiritual practice is simply this: Remember. Remember who you are. Remember what you love. Remember what is sacred. Remember what is true. Remember that you will die, and that this day is a gift. Remember how you wish to live."

– WAYNE MULLER, *HOW, THEN, SHALL WE LIVE?*

HILARY GREENSTREET:
FINDING CHOICES, FREEDOM, AND SELF

"Coming to Harmony Hill felt very much like visiting dear friends at their summer home. It wasn't just the amazing beauty of the setting; it was the warm environment, the caring people, the sense of complete safety. Everything we might have needed or wanted had been arranged for us, thoughtfully, from a private room and bath to teabags and hot chocolate."

Hilary Greenstreet's first impression of Harmony Hill was reinforced throughout her cancer retreat there in 2007. She had heard about the Hill through a cancer support group and went there at the conclusion of a brutal six months of surgery, chemo, and radiation. She went feeling completely depleted; her life no longer feeling as if it were her own.

Throughout her diagnosis and treatment, Hilary was continually reminded of all the things that had changed for her, all that she could no longer do – work out, go for walks, sleep through the night, and so on. In place of what she *couldn't* do, she was also told of all the things she now *must* do, including taking still more pills, going through frequent check-ups and testing, and visiting physicians and therapists several times each month.

"Freedom to make choices had been missing during my treatment. It was one 'have to' after another. I didn't have options.

"In treatment, you follow somebody else's plan for you. Even when that plan is in your best interest, it's hard to turn over your life that way; it takes away your sense of self, of who you are. You just keep putting one painful foot in front of the other, doing what others tell you to do, but you lose your independence and become increasingly dependent on the judgment of others."

When Hilary and her husband arrived at Harmony Hill, they were handed a schedule, and told that they didn't have to do anything on it unless they wanted to.

"We could do whatever we wanted to do, and not do whatever we didn't want to do. As it happened, we chose to participate in almost all the activities, but we were given the incredible freedom of knowing it was our choice.

"At Harmony Hill, you begin to make choices about your life again. That may sound small, but it felt huge, and wonderful. As cancer survivors, we started talking, exploring, thinking about all the things we *could* do, and the things that maybe we couldn't do quite yet but would soon be able to do again, all the things we had been missing. At the Hill, my focus readjusted to what I could do for myself, and even what I could possibly do for others.

"Slowly I was becoming aware of the many aspects of my life which *hadn't* changed because of cancer, all the things that I still could do, and the things that soon I would be able to do again. When I left, it was with the excitement and joy of feeling I had my life back."

Hilary was inspired by her fellow retreat participants: "We shared our stories, often in detail, but it wasn't a 'pity party.' It was relaxed and comfortable, safe and informative. There were powerful stories of courage and gratitude, as well as simple stories, offering help for some of the immediate difficulties we were facing. It meant so much to see people around me meeting the challenges in their lives, with profound grace, humor, and generosity. They spoke of some of the same struggles I was facing, and of some even greater challenges than those which confronted me. Their stories helped me immeasurably, and I can only hope my story might have helped someone else."

For part of the retreat, the cancer survivors and their caregivers met separately.

"This gave both groups the opportunity to say what was true, what we needed to say without feeling any need to protect our partners. It was safe to say exactly what was real without any need for sugar-coating harsh realities.

"For me, Harmony Hill was all about having a safe rebirth. My old personality came back, and with it came some new perspectives. There were new, wonderful things which had been added to my life, and there were some less-positive thoughts and ideas which I chose not to hang on to, not to allow back into my life. Before cancer and Harmony Hill, I tended to be somewhat self-conscious and judgmental about my every perceived flaw. After this experience, most of those 'problems' had disappeared, replaced by an intense sense of gratitude and, hopefully, some more meaningful values.

"I also made the decision not to waste my time with negative people. I always used to be the 'good girl,' the rule-abider, accepting whatever nonsense people dished out, not wanting to rock the boat. I find now I'm less tolerant of unkindness or bigotry – I'll go elsewhere. I'll bypass negativity and choose a positive route instead. I want to spend my energy and time with people I appreciate and enjoy. I'm now acutely aware that the time one has really is finite, and I find myself asking, 'Is this how I want to spend my time, spend my life?'"

Harmony Hill and the experience of cancer also renewed Hilary's interest in volunteering.

"So much had been given to me during the course of my treatment and at Harmony Hill that I felt a renewed motivation to give back. I began volunteering to teach ESL to non-native speakers, and I asked my family if they would be willing to forego buying me gifts for birthdays and Christmas, and instead, make donations to Harmony Hill."

"I'm not going to say that cancer was a blessing. Trust me: If I'd had a choice, I would not have chosen to have cancer. But cancer did force me to pause. Harmony Hill helped me to realize that I had been given an opportunity to step back and take another look at what I could do, what I wanted to do, and how I wanted to live my life. In short, I was given a rebirth.

"*Harmony Hill gently encouraged me to look to the future and let the past be past. I left Harmony Hill with a clear message: 'Now it's time to get on with the rest of your life.'*" ❖

By 2004, the number of scholarship requests for Harmony Hill cancer retreats had been increasing dramatically each year.

Recalls Gretchen, "We recognized that many, many individuals were not even contacting us because they could not afford to attend and were not comfortable asking for assistance. We did not want money to be a barrier to anyone having access to Harmony Hill. That's when the Board made the decision to offer our cancer retreats at no cost to participants."

As a result of this change, Harmony Hill found itself with waiting lists of people wanting to attend a cancer retreat. Based on funding available, nine retreats were scheduled for 2004. To provide interim support for those on waiting lists, the Hill inaugurated a one-day mini-retreat for those with cancer; it was called "Living with Cancer: Tools for the Journey." The one-day program – also free – offers practical resources and strategies such as guided imagery, nutrition, and simple movement, as well as useful information on how to live fully despite the challenges of cancer. While those on the waiting list for the three-day retreats are given first priority, the class is also offered to anyone with a cancer diagnosis who is interested. After experiencing the one-day "Tools" program, many of these individuals are eager to sign up for the three-day retreat. ❖

MICHELLE CLIFTON:
THE WAY ACROSS IS THROUGH

Michelle Clifton is a lucky woman. The tall, urbane redhead has it all: a beautiful career, family and home life. And when Michelle got cancer, she was lucky she got "Cancer Lite."

"I was about to celebrate my 41st birthday when I found the lump in my breast," she recalls. "I was so blessed that the lump was very small and close to my skin."

The medical decisions and processes, however, were extensive and drawn-out. Michelle agonized over the surgical choices she had to make, whether to reconstruct her breast and if so, whether the reconstruction should be done at the time of the mastectomy or after her body had had time to recover from the trauma of surgery before risking an implant.

"I was really scared all the way through. You're just sitting there in doctors' offices, and all these strangers are talking about *your life*, you know, talking about *statistics* and *your odds*."

She took her breast surgeon's advice and opted for the mastectomy, and decided to wait for the reconstruction. She lived without a breast for four months. It took another year and a half for the reconstruction, step by step and with some complications, to be completed.

"If I'd had that other surgery, I'd have woken up from the mastectomy with a boob, *bada-bing, bada-boom,* and just got back on the wheel. I've been a hairdresser my whole life, and being a hairdresser is all about your image, your appearance. For the first time in my life – going through my cancer – I really got it that I was more than my body. I never got that before."

What sustained her through it all? Without hesitation, Michelle answers, "My spirituality. I read every spiritual, personal-growth, self-help book I could get my hands on. I meditated, chanted, and I did a lot of chakra work, especially on my heart chakra."

Although she didn't have an "official" cancer support group, Michelle did have a lot of support while she was dealing with her cancer.

"I chose to share it with everybody, all my friends, family, and clients; I opened it up for others to give to me. My mother didn't share hers. She felt like her body betrayed her. A client of mine took a three-month sabbatical, took care of her cancer, then came back and didn't tell anybody. For me, I am glad I did it the way I did.

"Above all, I was so blessed to have my family. My partner Menno was always so loving and supportive through everything. He'd lost his mother to ovarian cancer just five years before I got mine. I felt so lucky to have had a breast removed and to be able to walk away and still feel like a beautiful woman – to still feel sexy, to keep my head high, and to be able to exude that energy.

"My youngest daughter, Aleana, who was only seven years old when I was diagnosed, was like a little angel. She wrote poetry as I was going through my cancer; she has a whole book of it.

"Feeling blessed to be on the planet after surviving my cancer, I had begun formulating an idea for a day retreat for women who have had breast cancer. A client of mine had been telling me about Harmony Hill and her friend Gretchen, who was the director. She encouraged me to visit, but I didn't do anything about it for a couple of years. The first time I went there was a gorgeous summer day in 2007."

That day, Gretchen and Michelle had a long chat about Michelle's retreat plans, and Gretchen invited Michelle to return to Harmony Hill for a "Tools for the Journey" workshop.

"Since my plan wasn't coming together the way I wanted it to, I thought, 'Okay, this workshop will be a good place to come and learn, to see how they do things here.'"

Michelle found the workshop to be a very humbling experience.

"Here I thought I was *way* past my cancer, my healing – that was all done; I was on this path to help others. I had all these ideas of how everything should be for my day retreat, what it would take to get people to open up. I was way off base.

"At the workshop, right out of the gate, I saw how *ready* people were to share. It's such a safe place; it's like this camaraderie thing – you're automatically safe. Everybody there is going through the exact same thing. You don't have to explain."

Yet when it came time for her to share in the group, Michelle found she could hardly speak.

"I felt very...small, somehow. I thought I was going to be this bright, shining light; I was going to have all this amazing stuff to share about how to get over your cancer. But when it came my time, the words did not come easy.

"I realized I still had some things to look at, that I was still healing, four years out from my bout with cancer. Maybe I had put the lid on it too soon. It's not something you just *get over*, you know, in time."

The three-day retreat was one of the "most real" experiences of Michelle's life.

"We don't get that opportunity in everyday life. People don't want to go that deep, it's too painful. But at Harmony Hill, that's what you're there to do: you're there to heal and to get face-to-face with how precious life is. To be able to do that was just amazing.

"The way the three-day retreat is planned, it's like it builds up to this crescendo during the time you have with the group. Hearts are open, everything is exposed. I don't think you can really go that deep in a once-a-week support group. You know, you drop your kids off before, and have to go home and make dinner afterwards. That's why those three days at Harmony Hill are so powerful – you're removed from everything, you're in these beautiful surroundings with all these people who are there for you. And the fact that it doesn't cost you any money, that's *huge*."

By their group's third meeting, Michelle discovered how powerful it is to "have people listen, I mean *really* listen to one another. There's no agenda, no place else to be, nothing else to do. They're really listening."

As Michelle listened, she felt guilty that her own cancer story "wasn't that bad," compared with the rest of the group.

"Listening to these women's stories just sort of broke my heart, and there I was – I'd never had chemo or radiation; I was, as I'd heard it put, totally 'cancer lite.'" By the end of the retreat, however, Michelle realized that "no matter what level of hardship one person encounters in another's story, cancer is cancer."

In 2009, Michelle hit the five-year survival mark. And still she keeps returning to Harmony Hill because, she says, "I'm just compelled; it's almost like I don't have a choice. In part I feel a responsibility because I've been so blessed. Before, I was a party girl, all about the party. The older I get, the more it's like, hey, it's really not about me. The way my journey's unfolded, it's made me look more deeply at everything. *I didn't go around anything, I went* through *it.*" ❧

> **❝The only way around is through."**
> – ROBERT FROST

GRETCHEN:
CANCER RETURNS...

In 2006, cancer returned. When I was diagnosed with follicular Non-Hodgkin's lymphoma, my first reaction was that I had failed. I had not beaten cancer back. Like every other cancer survivor, I had *so* wanted to be done with cancer, I had *so* wanted it to be ancient history. But it was back and I was depressed to be confronting a new round of treatment and more uncertainty. Also, like many cancer survivors who have a recurrence, I felt embarrassed and disappointed in myself. It's stupid to feel that way – I know that – but it's a common reaction: blaming yourself when, truly, it's something over which you have no control. As many times as I have seen that reaction among Harmony Hill retreat participants, and as many times as I have told them with all sincerity not to blame themselves or feel any guilt, I couldn't help having those feelings myself. Now it was my turn to listen to friends and my own inner wisdom and let go of any feeling that I did something wrong, let go of that feeling of *failure*.

In the face of this new diagnosis, my dear friends were again there for me. They told me they were pooling resources so I could go to Commonweal or attend a renewal retreat. Their generosity and kindness reduced me to tears.

In my meditations – which I have learned to trust greatly – I came to see that what I really needed was time in the warm blue-green waters of Kauai. My spirit yearned for the bright sunshine and vivid colors of the "garden island;" my body craved the warmth and the healing waters. So many wonderful friends donated the funds to make this healing trip possible, including first-class flights to and from the island paradise. Denise Carrico made a spectacular series of prayer flags adorned with bells and all the names of those who supported my journey. It was with me throughout the trip to Kauai and became a prominent symbol on our meditation table. While there, I had several Lomi Lomi massages, participated in support sessions with a small group of nurses (at a workshop Leonie Wolff was leading), and walked, walked, walked the beaches with my bare feet in the blue-green waters. I felt the heavy clouds of fear and failure lift from me and watched them evaporate into the rays of bright sunshine. I said a prayer of thanks every day for the many wonderful friends and family members who had made this trip possible and whose presence I felt with me constantly during this time of deep healing.

When I returned from this blessed respite, I felt stronger and ready to face whatever was ahead of me. I carried with me not just the heavenly renewal I had gained from Kauai, but the support and caring of so many wonderful friends who had made the trip possible.

Cancer still had more to teach me ... and I was ready to learn. I'd been down that path before so I knew it was doable. Being calm beyond the storm became my goal. ❖

> **"Even if our efforts of attention seem for years to be producing no result, one day a light that is in exact proportion to them will flood the soul."**
>
> – SIMONE WEIL

COBIE WHITTEN:
A PASSION AND A PRIVILEGE

Cobie Whitten never expected a place like Harmony Hill. She certainly never expected that it would become a very big part of her life.

Though she looks like a raven-haired heroine in a romance novel, Cobie is a health professional – a psycho-oncologist, a title which, she admits, sounds like "an oncologist gone whack-o." What her job actually entails is "looking at all the aspects of the cancer experience not subsumed under surgery, chemo or radiation," she explains. "We know that cancer can impact every aspect of your life: psychological, spiritual, financial, sexual, you name it. Psycho-oncology deals with the impact of diagnosis and the after-effects of the diagnosis. As a colleague of mine puts it, 'you may be cancer-free, but you're not free of cancer.' The impact of the disease can last for a very long time."

A psychology major in college, Cobie worked in a psych hospital as a tech for a year and then went on to grad school. She became interested in working with cancer patients when she connected with a mentor at the University of Illinois who was using cognitive behavioral techniques, such as hypnosis, with cancer patients to help treat nausea and vomiting. She got involved in the research group, and she was hooked.

Her dissertation on "The Psychological Adjustment to Uncertain Outcomes: The Threat of Cancer Recurrence" also provided invaluable experience for her.

"I learned a tremendous amount. I learned that it didn't matter about prognosis –

someone could have a great prognosis and still be worried sick, another person could have a very poor prognosis and be at peace. That was the very first time I had a hint about the difference between healing and curing.

"And this is something that has been absolutely reinforced in my days at Harmony Hill. You may be considered cured medically but you may not be healed, and you can be healed without being free of disease."

Cobie began working in the psycho-oncological field in her early twenties and had two kids "along the way."

"People would ask why I did this work. They'd often say, 'You must have a lot of cancer in your family.' And I'd say no.

"Well, we know that one in two men and one in three women will be diagnosed with cancer in their lifetime – staggering figures! I was naïve.

"Sure enough, my mom, a lifelong smoker, was diagnosed at age 75; she died three weeks after diagnosis. I was talking on the phone with her when she collapsed. She died while I was in the air flying from Seattle to Chicago. That was my first experience of having a close relative die of cancer. I had lost my dad (who died of a heart attack) when I was a college student. So losing my second parent, you know, even though I was in my late thirties...I felt like an orphan."

Some time later, Cobie and her husband divorced and both moved on to new relationships.

"One weekend he was in the DC area for work because he was going to get engaged to a woman who lived in the area. That weekend, at age 42 – when our kids were 9 and 14 – he found blood in his stool and went to the hospital emergency room. It turned out to be adenocarcinoma of the gastric esophageal junction, stage four, already in his liver. He got very aggressive treatment, which had pretty significant side effects. The kids spent time with him in late summer. It was really hard on both of them, especially my daughter.

"I tried to be honest about his prognosis and not give up hope but also not give them unrealistic expectations. He was diagnosed in March 2001 and died in January 2002. Now I had two children who were affected by the disease; our whole family was.

"A couple years later, one of my son's college application essay questions was 'As we get older we have to reluctantly discard things, what have you had to reluctantly discard?' My son, who was seventeen at the time, answered, *'my adolescent sense of immortality.'*

"Both my kids recognize life is precious and fragile, that no one knows what will happen tomorrow, and you really should not sweat the small stuff.

"When I first started this work, I'd ask the question, 'How do you live each day when faced with profound uncertainty?' I was so fascinated by that – intellectually fascinated by that. Now, having lived through these experiences has altered me profoundly and made me feel more at peace and less afraid. I'm not afraid to sit with people with cancer, with people close to death. I feel it's my passion and privilege to do this work. And Harmony Hill is an unbelievable gift to me and an incredible venue to share whatever I have to offer."

Cobie attended a one-day "Tools for the Journey" workshop with two oncology colleagues in 2008. She was "blown away" by the experience.

"At the beginning of the workshop, I was wondering, 'What is my role here? Am I an observer, am I a participant?' What was I thinking? Within 30 seconds, I was a participant! You cannot just observe. When we did one of the guided imagery exercises, we were very covered up and warm and cozy, and there was a crackling fire in the fireplace; we went through this exercise to surround ourselves with people we have loved and people who have loved us. One of mine was a college mentor who has since died; one of them was my Siberian husky dog; one was my husband. It was a very profound and moving experience for me, the recognition and realization during that exercise that those people are always with me. I think that's what leads me to be brave and less afraid – knowing that I am not alone, that they are always with me. And can be with me even more powerfully when I conjure them up to be. For me, that was just the quintessential Harmony Hill experience.

"I left transformed and feeling like I had found another home, and that's how I feel each time I'm there. Indeed, the first three-day retreat that I spent there, I needed Gretchen's guidance about how to return to my regular life. She suggested I walk the labyrinth. It turned out to be a bridging, transformative way to go back to 'the other side.' I had never had exposure to a labyrinth before the first Tools workshop. I think part of me used to be somewhat cynical, you know? You hear things and think, 'sure, yeah, right.'"

Now a faculty member and retreat facilitator, Cobie facilitates mostly three-day retreats.

"The first time I was there for a three-day retreat, I thought, 'I just met all these people yet I feel more connected to them than I do to most people in my life. Why is that? How is this different from if I was at a cocktail party or even at an academic retreat?' *It's because we all are acknowledging our humanity, our fear, our anxiety, our heart, our mortality. And, boy, once you start at that foundation, you can go to extraordinary places.*

"Most people live in a cave and the cancer kind of yanks you out of the cave – if you'll let it – and it's bright outside and scary and some people are still in the cave and they want you to come back in with them. But when you go to Harmony Hill, we're *all* out of the cave." ❖

"You've got to be willing to boogie with the bogeyman."

– GREGG LEVOY

AMBA AND DON GALE:
CHANGING THE CONVERSATION

Amba and Don Gale's home suggests well-travelled lives, spiritual focus, intellectual and artistic pursuits. It's a warm, open, joyful space they share with their thirteen-year-old daughter, Mariel. The peaceful, verdant setting by the water is a perfect spot for living and working: Amba is a transformational educator and coach, and Don has his own recording studio.

In the presence of this vibrant, delightful couple, it's hard to imagine them in a dark and fearful place. Yet there they were in February 1999, when Don was diagnosed with Stage 4 non-Hodgkin's lymphoma, peripheral B cell. It was a ravenous cancer. He went into the hospital and immediately began receiving huge amounts of chemotherapy, which was successful for the interim. At the same time, he and Amba began looking around for alternative options. They were referred to Harmony Hill by Commonweal and were able to get into a retreat two months after the initial diagnosis.

"We definitely needed a perspective that would give us a better, more resourceful relationship with cancer than we had," says Amba. "I knew I couldn't go on like I had been, so deep in fear I could hardly function. He was in better shape than I was."

"Well, I was holding my own," Don says. "And the two things I remember most about the Harmony Hill retreat were the food – highly nourishing and inspiring – and being able to talk with other people about death and dying. I found it was never satisfying to talk about this prospect of imminent death with someone who wasn't face to face with it themselves. Overall, I remember the feeling that I was not alone, and that was part of it – being able to feel like I was really communicating about this fear about death and dying. The freedom and lightness that conversation gave me when it dawned on me they *really knew* what I was talking about, that was something I'd never had before. It was a very intense and peaceful time.

"I also found the labyrinth a remarkable tool for self-reflection and for quieting my mind down when I needed to. There's an amazing energy around the redwood labyrinth; I walk it every time I'm out there."

"The retreat was just wonderful," Amba recalls. "It gave me what I needed in terms of being able to create room for myself to *be*. And it created 'room around the cancer,' as well. Rather than resisting the cancer, we were able to hold it as an opportunity. Or a gift."

The Gales also attended a second retreat, the one-day "Tools for the Journey" workshop, a year after their first one. The two became close friends with Gretchen Schodde, who supported them all the way through Don's cancer and helped connect them with practitioners as they explored alternative treatments – some of which were considered radical and didn't have a lot of credibility at the time.

"If Gretchen didn't know the answer to questions, she knew someone who did," says Amba. "We got really knowledgeable about food as medicine, antioxidants, acupuncture, the science behind being able to take care of the body while in such a harsh regimen of chemo. We just did everything, you know, full tilt boogie!"

Don agrees. "Everything I could see to do within my tolerance for activity, I did. The acupuncture was not the least among them. I felt a changed state in my body and in my consciousness *every* time I left there. It was amazing."

Don went through an incredible amount of chemo on his way, he hoped, to getting a stem cell transplant. He had eight months of CHOP ("I used to proudly be able to name and pronounce all of these chemicals in the acronym") chemotherapy in quantities "unknown to mortal man." And he did very well with it; his stem cells were harvested when it looked like he was free of the disease.

"CHOP made the cancer virtually disappear," Don says. "I say virtually because, ultimately, it didn't. I eventually qualified for the stem cell procedure, and I was in the hospital for three weeks. I did well with it and everybody thought there was a lot of 'hope.' They gave us a 50-50 chance for the CHOP and 50-50 for stem cell."

Neither treatment beat the odds, however, and as far as the doctors were concerned, there was nothing else they could do.

"The cancer came right back after the stem cell procedure. And the doctors' thinking is that if it comes back, it's the strongest cancer cells that survive the treatments, and now your whole cancer is made up of the strongest cells, so you've really got a diminished chance of getting through this.

"So they said, 'We'll make you comfy, make sure you're not in pain.' I had no idea at the time that this was a euphemism for, 'Go home and die, and we'll help you through it.' It never occurred to me that I was going to die, actually. There were some moments when I came face to face with that possibility, but in those dark hours when things weren't working, I was just thinking, 'Okay, what's the next thing I can find to get this to work?'"

Don told his doctors he wanted to try a new treatment he had heard about: Rituxin monoclonal antibody. At the time, it was an extremely radical treatment, and his doctors didn't want to give it to him. (Rituxin has since become a very important component of lymphoma treatment.)

"The Rituxin saved my life when I was a hair's breadth from kicking over. I had two, three, four weeks to live at the most, I think. And Rituxin stopped that temporarily, but with continued administration, it stopped it for three years. After the first treatment, the cancer was gone for a year, and when the cancer came back, they did the same treatment, which was good for another year. Then the cancer came back again, and after the third treatment, the cancer stopped growing, but didn't disappear. 'Aha!' I thought, 'the shine has gone off the silver bullet, so we'd better find something else.'

"I got a recommendation for a naturopath who specialized in cancer, and he started me on high-dose vitamin C for about six weeks. After six weeks, I had a CT scan and the cancer was gone. It never showed up again. I did that same vitamin C protocol two more times on my own, and since then, I just continue to take vitamin C. That was five or six years ago, and I consider that a cure. At the same time, I'm always aware that there's a potential for a recurrence, so I do what I need to do, in my opinion, to head that off. I eat a lot of veggies, drink green drinks, eat a lot of vitamin C and other supplements. In addition to diet and supplements, I think the ultimate cure came from changing my lifestyle, changing the way I thought, shedding some baggage. I make sure I don't get depressed for long periods of time...oh, and I make sure that I'm not fooling myself."

Amba joins in, "I want to say something about that [mindset]: we are affected by the conversations around us, and those conversations affect our spirit, our mind and our body. At a certain point we saw that the professional medical opinion around us was, basically, that the cancer could be managed, but ultimately it'll get him. We got to a place where we said to one another, 'We've got to find a doctor or a health professional who's very clear that the cancer is disappearable.' We take stands in this household," she says, smiling broadly. "And we were taking a stand for the cancer being disappearable.

"I think when people get cancer, they tend to get resigned; the fear gets to be too much. It's so gripping; it's easy to go into all sorts of automatic responses to fear, like denial, or just giving up. The principle, the commitment, is to being able to live a full life with the cancer while dealing with the cancer. I think that makes all the difference in the world. Getting freed up from the fear, it's just huge."

Don and Amba continue to be part of Harmony Hill, supporting its work and contributing to its mission. Amba books retreats for some of the graduate conversations that she leads at the Creekside building ("a healing, wonderful, awesome space.") Another way she likes to contribute is by offering partial or full scholarships for her leadership development training to Harmony Hill's staff members.

During their cancer retreat, Don and Amba stayed in the Lodge suite with a deck that looks over the arbor. When they made a naming donation to the Hill, they chose to name the arbor to honor Amba's parents (her mother died of ovarian cancer when Amba was a teenager; her dad passed away a few years ago from a stroke.) Their names, inscribed on a beautiful piece of agate, now forever grace the green-leafed entrance to Harmony Hill. ✿

> "It may be that when we no longer know what to do, we have come to our real work, and when we no longer know which way to go, we have begun our real journey."
>
> – WENDELL BERRY

MICHELE SHAPIRO:
WHERE THE HEART LEADS

"I know beyond a shadow of a doubt that people heal faster with support."

That's the belief that guides Michele Shapiro in the work that she feels called to do. She's been on Harmony Hill's Board of Directors since 2004, becoming president of the Board in 2006.

Before she "met the Hill," though, Michele lived and worked in her hometown of Los Angeles.

"I was working as an administrator for The Breast Care Center and The Oncology Center in Orange County. I had never worked in that specialty before; however, I had worked quite a bit at introducing alternative and complementary medicine into Western medical practices. And I had done a lot of reading about body-mind healing, books by people such as Bernie Siegel, Rachel Naomi Remen, Carolyn Myss, and Judith Orloff. One day, when I was having lunch with a friend, I drew up a business plan for a wellness center. We created a design and then I just put it away.

"When I was hired by the Breast Care Center, I found out the physicians were interested in support services and a body-mind-spirit approach. I then proposed to them that we build a wellness center adjacent to the cancer center, and I showed them my design. They already had a non-profit foundation that offered support and mentoring services to their breast cancer patients, so I became the liaison between their group and ours; and the support center was nearly finished by the time I left."

Michele was recruited to the Pacific Northwest for another medical administrative job in a different field, but her heart was still in cancer support. A friend took her to out to visit Harmony Hill and to meet Gretchen Schodde. They had a cup of tea, of course. Shortly thereafter she called to say she wanted to volunteer, and was asked if she'd like to help with a gardening project at Harmony Hill.

Well, Michele isn't a gardener; she doesn't really like to get her hands dirty, so she passed on that volunteer opportunity.

"Gretchen called back a half hour later," recalls Michele, "saying, 'No, no, we don't want you to volunteer in the garden! We want you on the Board!'"

At first, Michele was hesitant because she'd served on a board before, in L.A.

"That board was very political, and I didn't want to be on that kind of board again. But when I went to that first Harmony Hill Board meeting – just to check it out – I was blown away by their opening the meeting with a healing circle. I had never seen *that* before. The way this board functioned was the complete opposite of the one I'd been on before, and I wanted to be part of it."

One board event that Michele remembers with great fondness is the time they all wrote inspirational thoughts and wishes for healing on the subflooring during the construction of the Great Hall. It pleases her to know they're there, beneath everyone in the opening circle of each cancer retreat, below each person practicing yoga or tai chi, under every celebrant at the many festive occasions held in the Great Hall.

"I've learned so much from being part of Harmony Hill over the years: generosity, selflessness – especially from Gretchen – and philanthropy. I've learned a whole different mindset. From Lynne Twist (author of *The Soul of Money*), I discovered the true privilege of giving back. And Gretchen is so gracious; she really knows how to thank people, and that makes it a great pleasure to participate in the giving. Plus, there are such interesting and smart people who work there!"

It's gratifying for all Board members to know that they are contributing to the lives of so many people living with cancer, their families, their caregivers and their communities. For Michele, the memory of one specific person who attended a cancer retreat represents The Reason she works so hard to keep Harmony Hill growing.

"In my mind, the image of Emily Dade is perfectly clear, though she's been gone for some years now. She was just 32 years old, a wife and mother of two small children. She spoke at a concert fundraiser we held at Town Hall in Seattle. She looked beautiful in a simple black dress, standing there before 500 people. Her breast cancer had metastasized, she'd had a double mastectomy, and as I watched and listened to her, I remember feeling – with shock – that she was dying. She spoke so beautifully, so eloquently that evening. Emily's words and her spirit really touched me. I'll never forget her or that moment.

"I'll continue to be part of Harmony Hill, to be part of the family, in any role in which I'm needed. I'd like to see it grow into a bigger organization with more outreach. Because *a support group of peers – which is completely different than talking with one's friends – is absolutely essential to a person's healing,* whether it's from the experience of cancer or the stress of caregiving or the suffering of grief and loss." ❧

> **❝**The only way to make sense out of change is to plunge into it, move with it, and join the dance."
>
> – ALAN WATTS

JERI PRAUL:
INCENTIVE FOR CHANGE

Two weeks before her cancer diagnosis in 2002, Jeri Praul recalls saying of her high-stress job at Harborview Medical Center, "This job is killing me."

She remembered those words when she got her diagnosis. Jeri chose not to continue working during her treatment for breast cancer.

"I took the year off to take care of myself and to live consciously. I participated in cancer support groups, I did yoga, I ate well, rested, and exercised. I met some amazing people and found so much support. I went through treatment without a lot of side-effects, and I think all of these things helped."

"During that year of treatment," Jeri says, "I learned how to be fully present, to 'be here now' in every moment. Cancer was one of the best things that ever happened to me. It forced me to look at how I was living my life and to face the question of what I wanted to be doing. I realized I wanted to be more conscious about how I spend my time and who I spend my time with. That was a year of growth and understanding for me, and when I had an opportunity to go to Harmony Hill at the end of my treatment, I went totally open to whatever would come up.

"I wanted to discover what my 'new normal' was. It was time to think about going back to work, and I wanted to see how I could do that and also carry forward all that I had learned during that year. I thought Harmony Hill might help me figure out how to keep those feelings of presence and centeredness, help me answer the question, 'Now what?'"

Jeri wasn't disappointed. She went to the retreat with her partner, Joan.

"We noticed immediately how nurtured we felt. Harmony Hill is an amazing place. It's so easy to settle in and feel connected to the place and to the purpose: healing. It's a safe setting to allow yourself to own your feelings and see what comes up, and to see how to move forward with your life.

"At Harmony Hill, all the distractions have been removed. There's no television, no telephone. You have to be with yourself. You have to be quiet and listen to that little voice within you that you don't often hear."

One of her most vivid memories of her retreat was the experience of a "sound bath."

"Three of the faculty rang Tibetan bowls all around us as we lay on the floor after a yoga session. The sound created a warmth and vibration that fully enveloped me. It felt like my cells were rearranging themselves. It was incredible!"

Jeri left Harmony Hill with the tools and the resolve to move forward with the same awareness and self-care she had drawn on during her treatment. She initiated actions which eventually led to a new position at her hospital – one with regular hours and far less stress.

Jeri and Joan also knew when they left Harmony Hill that they wanted to find a way to stay connected to it. They were invited to return as housemothers. Since 2003, Jeri has been a housemother for cancer retreats at least once a year. She goes to be a part of the healing process for others, but always finds something unexpected for herself.

"Every time I come to Harmony Hill, I touch that quiet place inside of me, and, without trying, I always gain clarity about some issue I've been working on."

Having been through the experience of both cancer and the Harmony Hill retreat helps her to be a supportive housemother for others taking the journey. Jeri notes, "I think of myself as staying behind the scenes, silently anticipating their needs, with the intent of helping them to have just the retreat that each of them needs. It always amazes me to see the transformation in each participant between Friday afternoon and the time they leave on Sunday - the shift from fear, anger, and sadness to joy and hopefulness. It's a wonderful thing to witness."

Jeri feels that the skills she employs as a housemother combined with the lessons she learned from her own cancer experience have helped her to be a better nurse: "Before cancer, I protected myself from uncomfortable situations. Now, I'm more open, more grounded, I'm able to be comfortable and present for others - no matter what they may be going through."

Cancer has also become a yardstick to maintain perspective. When Jeri and Joan are faced with troubling situations, they say to themselves, "How bad is it really? It's not cancer," which usually reminds them the problem is not worth spending a lot of time worrying about. It also reminds them how much they have to be grateful for.

"It is a privilege to be connected with Harmony Hill. Gretchen has created this amazing place. She had the vision and the ability to make it happen. Like Gretchen herself, Harmony Hill is calm and centered, caring and nurturing, and able to make you comfortable instantly. Harmony Hill helps each of us discover how to live our lives differently, how to live more fully." ❖

**"If you asked me
what I came in this
world to do, I will tell
you: I CAME TO
LIVE OUT LOUD."**

– EMILE ZOLA

ROGER DAY:
HOW YOU SPEND YOUR LIFE

Roger Day lost his wife, Karen, to lung cancer that had metastasized to her brain and heart. Karen had learned about Harmony Hill through an Internet search, but was too sick to be able to attend the retreat she had signed up for.

Only about six months after Karen's death, Roger was diagnosed with early prostate cancer.

"Mine was detected very early, so I was a candidate for 'watching and waiting,' he says, "but I had just lost my wife to cancer; I wasn't going to sit around waiting for anything. I decided on a procedure at the Seattle Prostate Institute, whose seed implants have a good success rate. They're kind of pioneers in that procedure."

Roger got a call from his friend, Ann Lovejoy. "She told me a cancer workshop was starting the next day and suggested I call Gretchen to see if I could get in. I called and in less than 24 hours I was at the retreat."

During the three-day retreat – which he attended alone – Roger found, "There's real value in people coming together as patients and caregivers to share what it's like. It's a good, safe place for them to express anger or sadness or whatever they're feeling. I could see it gave people permission to take more charge of their own life instead of leaving it up to their doctors. That's a hard one, it's so reinforced."

"It would have been great if Karen and I could have gone through that program together while she was alive. You know, it's funny, you always think you say everything you want to say but you realize afterwards – at least for me afterwards, there are other things you wish you'd talked about or done or said that you just don't do."

Reflecting on his Harmony Hill experience, Roger describes what he finds most important in life.

"It comes down to asking yourself this: *'How do you spend your time, your energy, your money? How do you use your time with the people who love you and the ones you love?'"* ❧

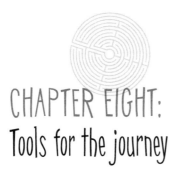

CHAPTER EIGHT:
Tools for the journey

"Cancer does not choose its victims according to 'ability to pay.' So much of the care and treatment, however, does depend on that. Being given care at no charge, regardless of 'ability to pay' works magic for those who cannot pay, and for those who can. Being given, free of charge, the love, respect and nurturing, made me feel worthy. For that reason, I have become a monthly supporter of the Hill." – BRENDA BISCIGLIA

While the cancer retreats are the core of Harmony Hill's mission and purpose, over the years many additional programs have been added to help fund the cancer programs and to offer opportunities for renewal, reflection, and healthy living.

Fee-based programs have included yoga, nutrition, labyrinth orientation, cooking, gardening, Tai Ji, healthy lifestyles, and several programs designed to provide renewal for nurses and other health professionals. Each year, the Hill offers more programs that connect it to the community and introduce more people to the magic that is Harmony Hill.

Harmony Hill is also available to outside groups looking for a special location for a meeting or retreat. Currently, it can offer sleeping accommodations for 35 people and meetings facilities for up to 160. It's been the site of many celebrations, including weddings, anniversaries, and family reunions.

More and more, the Hill is also welcoming individuals who are seeking a peaceful place for personal retreats. It's a place to rest and renew, to stroll the gardens, hike the surrounding hills, gaze at the breathtaking view of the Hood Canal and Olympic Mountains, or curl up by the fireplace with a good book. Nurtured by the surroundings and the kitchen's bounty, guests leave feeling replenished and already looking forward to their return. ❧

VOICE nurses

As Harmony Hill's retreats for people living with cancer evolved, Gretchen envisioned a parallel path for the healing professionals who care for them and others struggling with illness. Just as Harmony Hill provided a healing place for people with cancer, why couldn't it do the same for nurses and other health care providers?

Among the many health care professionals who have partnered with Harmony Hill over the years – to facilitate retreats, offer special programming, and contribute countless hours as volunteers – is a group of seven nurses, including Gretchen herself. Originally connected through their service as "house mothers" for cancer retreats, they came together a few years ago with the collective vision of creating healing programs for health care professionals. They recognized from their own experiences and from interactions with colleagues that nursing and other health care careers could be stressful, wounding and, at times, depleting.

They called themselves the VOICE (Vision, Opportunity, Inspiration, Compassion and Education) for Healers in Healthcare. Together they sought to inspire the transformation of the health care culture and to promote healing for people and the health professionals who care for them. Their mission was to offer educational and personal growth opportunities for reconnecting health professionals with the healing spirit of their work. They developed two programs for nurses at any stage in their careers.

"Creating Nursing Community: Your Story as a Healing Path" is a one-day program based upon the work of Rachel Remen, MD, Founder and Medical Director of Commonweal, the Northern California-based cancer program that inspired Harmony Hill. Dr. Remen's work on the healing power of story is the foundation of this program, offering nurses the opportunity to share their stories in a safe and supportive environment, and to experience what Remen refers to as generous listening. Attendees are also provided the tools to create their own story circles once they return home, as a way of building and sustaining the kinship of nursing.

"It's also about forming community," says Linda Covert, RN, one of the VOICE nurses.

"The experience of nurses being listened to by other nurses creates a transformation. Being acknowledged is a powerful thing. There's a woundedness in most of our lives. If we can touch that in a safe place, it opens us up to powerful healing."

"Most caregivers never have a chance to tell their stories," adds Kathlene Tellgren, RN, CEN, HN-BC, another of the VOICE nurses. "Doing so activates both the power of *intention* and *attention*." Where we place our attention molds us and defines who we are. When we're sharing our stories, we're acknowledging our intentions. "It's not about fixing, not about right or wrong. It's about the journey and the healing power of telling our stories and listening generously to the stories of others. It's about embracing our own wisdom."

VOICE nurse Leonie Wolff, RNC, LMT, notes that, "At first, we struggled to see how we could offer this program – what format, what sort of foundation...? One day we realized that we were creating the program we envisioned through living and sharing our own lives, and we saw that at the heart of healing is the telling of our stories."

"Embracing the Wisdom of Nursing" is a three-day workshop developed by Leonie Wolff. This program honors the hearts and hands of nurses and the very personal and intimate work they do. It explores concepts such as loving-kindness, grace, compassion, dignity, and generosity of spirit. Through stories, movement, art, and experiential activities, nurses are supported, inspired, and rejuvenated.

The program provides a space in which nurses can discover who they are in all their wholeness and all their beauty. For three days, they are encouraged to let go of the stresses of their jobs – the patient care, the paperwork, and the obligations. They are given the opportunity to rest and be cared for and nurtured. Cradled in a beautiful and comfortable setting, with delicious, wholesome meals provided, they have permission to just *be*. In essence, they experience *receiving* that which they so often give to others.

The retreat uses many of the same tools as the cancer workshops. It opens in circle; participants share their stories throughout. Movement, music, art, and the labyrinth offer means for nurses to experience their wholeness and to explore and express their personal journey, as well as their career path and vision for their own future.

They come away with a profound understanding of their own healing capacities, as well as new levels of connection to their chosen fields, and their personal sense of purpose.

"I don't think we knew it at the time," says Linda Covert, "but when we came together as the VOICE nurses, we were creating the community we needed to sustain ourselves, as much as we were crafting a program to help other nurses.

"Being a nurse is not just a job, it's heart-work. And when nurses come together and tell their stories, when they're listened to and acknowledged by their peers, it's a powerful reinforcement and validation."

"So many of us find that the pain of caring so much leads to burnout," adds Kathlene Tellgren. "We learn early on to armor ourselves against all of this, against all that we're carrying – the losses, the grief we're holding, the struggles we're witness to. Instead of closing ourselves, if we can become more open, we create that place for a healing encounter – for ourselves and for others.

"As nurses, when we see pain and suffering and grief, our inclination is to want to carry it. But what we offer through these programs is the vision that, instead, we carry *ourselves* with honor and strength, and then we're able to support others as they go through their pain."

In coming together as the VOICE nurses, these seven women formed a community that each of them needed. They provided support and compassion for one another through career changes, personal losses, and serious illness.

"We gave voice to what we intended," says Linda. "Through this community, it's become crystal clear to me that my goal, my mission, is to encourage and mentor young nurses in my daily work."

Linda recalls a recent experience of helping a young nurse deal with the first death she encountered professionally: "I made it a point to be with her throughout the process. I stayed with her, provided some guidance, answered her questions, and talked to her after her patient died. I checked in with her during the day and at the end of her shift. I encouraged her to feel what she was feeling and to express it, not to bury it. She was so appreciative of my presence and support, and I knew she would be equipped to handle the next death she faced. That's what VOICE does – supports nurses to do the incredible work we do, and to do it in a way that keeps us whole.

"Healing means bringing wholeness. If we can support nurses to do this extraordinary work and to find a place where they can remain whole in nursing, we will be doing our own heart-work." ❖

> **"**To be human is to become visible while carrying what is hidden as a gift to others."
>
> – DAVID WHYTE

DENISE CARRICO:
TRANSFORMING BODY AND SPIRIT

Denise Carrico – talented, caring, spirited, creative and generous – is a gem at the heart of Harmony Hill.

Denise has been teaching yoga for twenty-three years, beginning on the East Coast, mostly on the North Carolina Outer Banks. In 1997, when she moved to Seattle, she found a position substituting for a woman who was teaching a Yoga-for-Cancer class for Cancer Lifeline.

"That class really spoke to the style of yoga that I wanted to teach; it informed and transformed the way I teach. All of this work has changed my own practice, my own way of viewing a yoga practice and certainly my way of teaching, whether a cancer class or a regular class."

Shortly after she took the part-time position, Denise was teaching two classes on a regular basis. The classes got larger and larger as people living with cancer discovered that yoga made them feel better, more peaceful, even if it was only for that ninety minutes of class. One couple (the husband living with cancer) found Denise's class so vital they made a very large donation that allowed Cancer Lifeline to add yet another class.

"At the time, there were probably only two of us in Seattle who were teaching yoga classes specifically for people living with cancer. Even today, thirteen years later, there aren't many who offer what we do. "

Denise had been teaching at Cancer Lifeline for about a year when a serendipitous friend-of-a-friend's referral led Denise to Harmony Hill. Melissa West, a woman Denise had never met, called to ask Denise if she would like to apply for the position of movement teacher at a place she'd never heard of, Harmony Hill.

"In fact, she asked if I wanted to apply *and* to teach a yoga workshop for their upcoming cancer retreat the very next weekend!" Denise recalls with a laugh. "Though I'd never done anything like this before, I went."

Denise was hired that weekend, and she met Gretchen for the first time.

"I'll never forget what Gretchen said to me that weekend when we first met," Denise recalls. "She said 'It feels like you have always been here but now you've just shown up.'"

Denise found that teaching yoga at the Harmony Hill cancer retreats was a very different experience from teaching her 90-minute classes.

"Being with a group for a weekend is just phenomenal," she says. "Though we only have an hour of practice, we meet four times during the retreat, so there is some continuity, and I try to make it somewhat sequential.

"Psychotherapist Sharon Saltzman talks about what happens in the room in the relationship between therapist and client that makes it a momentous thing. She says, 'It's not what I say, recommend or suggest; it's not anything I *do* in particular. It's the love in the room.' I think about that a lot, especially when we're sitting in the cancer retreat's first circle Friday with a new group. I'll think, 'Oh, these people don't have a clue yet...just wait until Sunday when we come back again and sit in this circle!' And come Sunday, you just see it in their eyes – they're in love with each other, they're just totally in love!

"It's life-changing; you come into this group with 19 or 20 strangers and you leave with a family. Like with yoga, even in one day it happens – when you leave, you know someone better, you've made some kind of connection."

While still teaching classes in the Seattle area at the YMCA, 8 Limbs Yoga, and Cancer Lifeline, as well as facilitating yoga at the Harmony Hill cancer retreats, Denise began offering wellness yoga workshops at Harmony Hill in 2003.

"I started doing some of these workshops on my own – the women's annual weekend retreat (in May) and the Grace & Gratitude workshop (in November), and I've continued them because people really like them. These workshops are offered for a fee, which helps to support the mission of Harmony Hill – to continue to offer, free-of-charge, one-day and three-day cancer retreats."

People love doing yoga with Denise, and many of her students have been practicing regularly with her for years. She encourages each individual to practice at whatever level his or her own body allows, to focus on the breath, to find the strength and peace at one's core, and to celebrate spirit, body and community. And at the end of each workshop, there are small, meaningful gifts for all, handcrafted by the artistic yogi herself: favorite quotes and poems, a shell or bookmark embellished with her exquisite calligraphy, a heart-shaped stone.

In 2010, after four or five years' talking about the possibility, Denise moved from her West Seattle home to Harmony Hill to take on the full-time role of Caretaker. Living on the grounds, Denise is there when staff is not available to greet retreat participants and visitors, to give people tours, to lighten Gretchen's load, to maintain the labyrinth ("It feels holy to me, it's my way of walking it"), and to coordinate Night Watch volunteers to cover her caretaking duties when she must be away from the Hill. Living on the grounds has also allowed her to offer weekly yoga classes at Harmony Hill to local residents, as well as to visitors.

"Eventually, I'd love to see other faculty living here, perhaps a Harmony Hill intentional community. I feel kind of like the guinea pig. I'm the first of many, I hope.

"Thinking back to when I first arrived at Harmony Hill, the feeling was *'this is the beginning of something great!'* Thirteen years later it's still here, I'm here, and it's just amazing!" ❖

The following poem (an excerpt from one of Denise's favorite poets) was written on the wall behind the refrigerator of her new Harmony Hill apartment as a surprise "welcome" blessing:

For a New Beginning

Though your destination is not yet clear
You can trust the promise of this opening
Unfurl yourself into the grace of beginning
That is at one with your life's desire

Awaken your spirit to adventure
Hold nothing back, learn to find ease in risk
Soon you will be home in a new rhythm
For your soul senses the world that awaits you

– JOHN O'DONOHUE

DIANNA BLOM:
A PLACE TO RELAX AND FIND MY CENTER

Dianna has been a nurse for more than 40 years. She's been coming to Harmony Hill as a house-mother since 2003. There are generally two nurse "housemoms" at every cancer retreat. They don't sit in on the entire program, but they're there to help and support facilitators in some of the programs, to tend to any medical needs that may arise for attendees, and to be a safe person to talk to at any time, day or night.

Herself a breast cancer survivor, Dianna is someone participants know they can come to and she will understand what they're going through.

"I feel privileged to be there. Hearing people's stories and seeing them change during the course of the weekend, witnessing their courage and willingness to be open, watching friendships form – it often feels miraculous."

Harmony Hill's mission and commitment to not charging for the retreats assures a welcome diversity that contributes to the magic. Says Dianna, "At a single retreat, there may be ages ranging from 20s through 70s, CEOs, physicians, or laborers. And once they're here, they connect in a deep and meaningful way, no matter what their background. Those connections – that's where the magic is."

Dianna is often moved by the courage of attendees, by their willingness to be open and vulnerable over the course of three days among strangers. She particularly remembers Barbara Oswald, who never let the fact that she was blind deter her from fully experiencing Harmony Hill.

"She touched us all. She was so articulate about who she was; she spoke from her true, authentic self and from a place of deep joy. She was very independent, but she could also be vulnerable and accepting of help if it was offered. Her spirit heart was wide open and it was inspiring to be in her presence."

Dianna is one of the founding members of VOICE for Healing in Healthcare. She is also a certified Cross-Cultural Music in Healing Practitioner, Therapeutic Touch Practitioner, and a graduate of the Spirituality, Health and Medicine program at Bastyr University. She is passionate about sharing these gifts with her nursing colleagues and retreat participants. She marvels at the changes she's seen happen to people through sound, story, movement, labyrinths, and the great variety of activities offered at Harmony Hill.

"It has all the tools in the toolbelt. One size does not fit all, but there is something there for everyone to help put them in touch with their authenticity, with their heart. When you come from your truth, the right thing will happen. It always does.

"For me, Harmony Hill is a place to relax and to center. When I'm there, amidst the peacefulness and the amazing natural setting, it feels as if I've come home to myself." ❧

TED SPEAKMAN:
GROWING WITH THE HILL

Ted Speakman has been involved with Harmony Hill – in a variety of ways – since the earliest years, when there was just a house, garage, and small mobile home that served as Gretchen's residence. He was working at Fred Hutchinson Cancer Research Center when he was asked to visit the Hill to consult on a new phone system. He was accompanied on the visit by his partner, Vern, and both felt the magic of Harmony Hill as soon as they stepped onto the property.

"It's the same today as it was then. As soon as you drive up the hill, it's like you're in another world. You feel the peace of the place, and there's an immediate release of bad energy."

Vern hit it off with Gretchen right away and became a volunteer. In the early days, there were always projects for his handyman skills – plumbing, carpentry, working in the garden or the kitchen. If Gretchen thought of something the Hill needed, Vern said he could do it...and he did. Pretty soon, Vern was living at Harmony Hill, working as facilities manager, and Ted came out to stay on weekends.

Ted and Vern participated in a variety of fundraising activities for the Hill, but their favorite was decorating Christmas trees for the homes or businesses of large donors. Each tree was a stunning and customized holiday treasure, some garnering as much as $4000 for Harmony Hill.

Whenever a cancer retreat was scheduled, Vern was there to help with the set-up and anything that participants might need. He took seriously the job of making sure the Hill looked perfect when people arrived. He often sat in on parts of the retreats, and if Ted was there, he would join in, as well. They learned yoga and meditation; they learned about nutrition and how to live more healthfully. Like the retreat participants, they came away with a better understanding of self-care and a sense of spiritual connection. Ted describes it as "a spiritual awakening – spiritual not in a religious sense, but in a way that you feel the energy of life, you become aware that how you choose to live each day moves you forward physically, mentally, emotionally, and spiritually."

"When we do what we love, again and again, our life comes to hold the fragrance of that thing."

– WAYNE MULLER

Neither suspected at the time they were participating in the cancer retreats that they would be touched by the disease themselves. Vern was diagnosed with lymphoma in 2002, and died only a few months later, not directly of cancer but from a virulent infection. A celebration of his life was held on the property, and a rose bush blooms there in his memory. Ted was diagnosed with kidney cancer in 2006 and successfully treated for the disease. Gretchen and the Hill provided spiritual and emotional support for both of them. They also benefited from all they had learned over the years at Harmony Hill.

Two long-term takeaways for Ted have been meditation and nutrition.

"I didn't even know what meditation was before I visited Harmony Hill. It's become an important part of my life. I've learned how to quiet busy thoughts and go with the flow. Even today, I meditate for an hour each day, and I don't get caught up in all the negative energy that surrounds us or bombards us from the media. Meditation centers and grounds me."

Eating well has also become a big part of Ted's life. He loves to cook and uses the Harmony Hill cookbook and healthy eating tips he learned at the Hill.

"The food there was always so good. We learned how to eat healthy and how to cook wonderful meals without sugar, white flour, and other harmful ingredients. I still cook that way. I'm 62 years old, but I feel like I'm 35."

Ted has been on the Harmony Hill Board of Directors for many years. He looks back in awe at how far the Hill has come.

"Being a part of Gretchen's vision and making it all come true has been a privilege. Watching it grow and offer more programs and serve more and more people ... I just wish everyone knew about Harmony Hill."

"Vern and I were both deeply touched by Harmony Hill. It made us better people, more caring and more understanding, better able to handle all we went through. I feel like I'm a changed person. I'm more aware of life and of my surroundings. Every day, I think about what else I'm here to do. There's a saying that Disneyland is the most magical place on Earth. Me? ... I'd rather go to Harmony Hill." ❖

❝ He who sows sparingly will reap sparingly, and he who sows bountifully will reap bountifully."

– ST. PAUL

Kore Leadership is one of several organizations that use Harmony Hill's facilities for retreats and a variety of other programs. Since 2005, the Hill has been the setting for Kore's public and corporate workshops and retreats designed for women from business, medicine, law, government, and the arts – women who desire to lead in ways that bring all of themselves to what they do, and, in so doing, change the world. Suzanne Anderson, Founder and President of Kore Leadership, notes that the physical setting first drew her to the Hill.

"It's exceptionally beautiful and magical. The gardens and buildings all reflect the incredible care and love of so many people. The staff at Harmony Hill are exemplary in their care and generate a special atmosphere that is very healing and nurturing."

Beyond that, Suzanne also saw early on that executive director Gretchen Schodde's style of leadership "is absolutely aligned with our work. Gretchen is a model who has realized her calling to create a retreat center where people could experience renewal and deep well-being. We are dedicated to the education and support of those who are ready to be the change they want to see in the world. We've been coming to Harmony Hill for years now and will continue to think of it as a sacred setting for our retreats." ❧ ❧

MARTHA PHILL:
IT'S ALL ABOUT ATTITUDE

Martha Phill has spent a lot of time on the Hood Canal; her father built the family's summer house there in 1949. Years later, when Martha's own five children were grown and beginning families of their own, a nurse named Gretchen Schodde moved onto a nearby property on the Canal. Martha was curious to meet her.

"The first time I met her, about 20 years ago, she made such an impression. After a while, everybody on the Canal knew Gretchen. She was 'The Nurse.' If anyone had any kind of problem, she would get called, and she would come down and rescue or help us. She was so amazing, always planting and digging, growing the gardens. They would build one nice cabin up there on The Hill, then another; they would hold yoga classes, have seminars. I remember when they built the labyrinth – that was so interesting! I always wanted to see more of Gretchen than I did."

Martha would have the opportunity to get to know Gretchen and Harmony Hill much better. In 1999, at age 70, she was diagnosed with lung cancer. She'd had an aggravating pain for quite a while that wasn't going away, but since there was no history of cancer in her family, both Martha and her doctor were shocked. Her doctor opted to take the whole lung out, instead of risking more surgeries. Martha had always been healthy and athletic – hiking, biking, running, doing aerobics every day, so she was in good shape for surgery and optimum post-op healing.

"I was one of the lucky ones; I didn't have to have chemo or radiation. My doctor was wonderful. It still amazes me when I think about it: the scar is only a few inches long under my arm."

Martha didn't go to Harmony Hill right away, she says, because "back then their emphasis was on breast cancer."

Then, in 2000, cancer was found in one of Martha's breasts.

"The doctor decided, due to my age, mostly, to take the whole breast. It was on the same side where my lung had been removed, so afterwards I really felt *lopsided*," she recalls with a laugh. "But I just thought, 'I'm gonna deal with this,' and I did, with no reconstruction."

With the diagnosis of breast cancer, Martha figured it was her time to go to Harmony Hill. She went to talk with Gretchen, and signed up for the next three-day cancer retreat.

Martha's face lights up as she recalls those three days: "It was wonderful! It was the first time I'd ever taken part in meditation. Someone there did Reiki, and it was thrilling. I could really feel the transfer of healing power from their hands to my body. The group leaders were a psychologist and his wife; they were very good at helping us find the way to say how we felt.

"Many of these people had not been able to share their feelings with anybody else; they were just *hungry* to get some support. Some of them, their family members wouldn't even say the word 'cancer.' I got tremendous support from my family, but it's never been real easy for me to share private things. A lot of people aren't used to sharing emotions like that. But if you kept it in the family, kept it to yourself, you'd never realize that others are hurting just as much as you are.

"But you get in this circle and you find out people are caring about what you're saying, and maybe there's somebody who felt the same way you do, and you just want to blurt out, 'Oh, yes! That's the way I feel, too, and that's what I want to say, too!' It makes you feel good that someone else thinks the same way, and that you're not crazy." She laughs heartily.

"And I think that *once you've got it out of your mouth, you're already on your way to healing.*

"There were a lot of emotions, and I don't want to paint too sad a picture because there was humor there, too. We had some people who would share something funny that happened to them because of their cancer. Everybody could laugh because maybe it happened to them and they couldn't see the humor in it before, but now they could. That's one thing that really did impress me: *Isn't this wonderful? We are laughing!* It was easier to laugh, of course, when you were in this group with others in the same boat.

"They also have retreats at Harmony Hill that the caregivers and families of people with cancer can attend. My husband died of brain cancer when he was only 55; I took care of him for two years at home, so I'd had some knowledge of how awful this disease is before I got it myself. And I did a lot of things then that I would have done differently now.

"Being at Harmony Hill gives you a good attitude. You find out some of the people who have the worst cancers and worst treatments have the most positive attitudes. I learned there that attitude makes such a difference.

"Oh, and the food! You can't say enough about the food at Harmony Hill. They stress good eating habits there, and all the food is organic and so delicious and so comforting."

Actually, Martha can't say enough about Harmony Hill and Gretchen Schodde. "After you've been there, you just want to share all this with everybody." ❖

> "Our attitude towards what has happened to us in life is the important thing to recognize.... The last of human freedoms, to choose one's attitude in any given set of circumstances, is to choose one's own way."
>
> – VICTOR FRANKL

MAROLAN TILCOCK:
HERE FOR A REASON

There's something angelic about Marolan Tilcock: her sapphire eyes, her sweet smile and calm, gentle voice. The way she glows when she talks about her husband, her daughter, her grandmother. She's also very grounded, funny and earthy. But Marolan has been through hell, a journey through which she forged an intimate relationship with angels.

When Marolan's first marriage was disintegrating, she took her baby girl, Hannah, and went to visit her family in Texas for a break from the turbulent relationship. Along with the emotional stress, Marolan also knew that something was physically wrong with her; she had what she thought were all the symptoms of a bad bladder infection. She went to the emergency room, where the doctor did an internal exam and said she needed to get in to a gynecologist immediately.

The next day she went to a clinic where the doctor assured Marolan there was no need to worry, that the possibilities of there being anything serious were miniscule. Her pelvic exam, unfortunately, revealed a different story. The doctor could *see* the tumor, and he put a rush on the pathology tests.

The kind of cervical cancer that Marolan was diagnosed with is very rare and very aggressive. In the nine years since her diagnosis, Marolan has never met a fellow survivor, only the friends and family of those who have died from it.

Within five days of her diagnosis, Marolan was rushed in for a full hysterectomy and lumpectomy. The surgeons removed thirty lymph nodes from her pelvis, an extremely painful excavation from which it took three long months to recover. During her recuperation, her marriage proved to be beyond reconciliation. It was a long, hard road to recovering both her physical and her emotional health.

Four and a half years later, Marolan's life was going well. Her divorce and her bout with cancer were behind her. She bought her own condo. She became an administrative assistant at Microsoft. She loved her job, and there she met Alex, who would eventually become her life partner. Two weeks before Christmas 2004, Alex surprised Marolan with a proposal to marry while they were visiting her parents' ranch. While in Texas, Marolan's back was giving her a good deal of pain and was growing worse.

When she returned home and went back to work, Marolan was in such pain she couldn't sit at her desk. Not for one moment did it ever occur to her that it was her cancer, but an MRI revealed that it had returned. It was wrapped around her sciatic nerve, squeezing it "like a balloon" and the pain had become excruciating.

Doctors started her on an IV of dilaudid for the pain and kept her on it for a year and a half. They began chemotherapy, but it was the wrong cocktail and Marolan became violently ill. The joy of the wedding was short-lived. Marolan's condition was worse than she knew; Alex went from being a newlywed to becoming a caretaker, and Marolan's mother put her own life on hold as she moved in to help provide round-the-clock support for the family.

Over time, Marolan slowly began to get better. And finally, with the right formulations and combinations of therapies, she went into remission in the spring of 2006.

Just three short months after remission, the cancer came back. It wrapped around her spine and was woven within her peridium muscle and her sacrum. This time, her doctor told her she was terminal, and there was nothing more he could do for her. So Marolan went to a new doctor at Seattle Cancer Care Alliance. At their first meeting, Marolan asked him just one question: "Do you think you can put me in remission?"

His immediate response: "Of course I can!" That was all she wanted to hear.

At this point, Marolan had a great deal of radiation damage. There were holes throughout her colon, and her hips were disintegrating. She had ninety rounds of five-hour hyperbaric treatments to get her colon working. This time, Marolan says, "I was willing to do every single thing I had to do to get well, no matter what."

The first time she was diagnosed, Marolan knew she had to *get well* for her two-year-old daughter. The second time, Marolan knew she had to *live* for Hannah, but the third time, she says, "I knew I had to live for me, that *I had to find myself worthy to live*, and that was really hard for me."

When her acupuncturist asked Marolan what she thought about healers, about going to someone who called herself "an angel healer," Marolan said, "Bring it on!

"I really didn't know what to think, but I was willing to try *whatever* and to keep an open mind. And the session was *amazing*. I didn't know if it healed me or not; I just thought of it as a most amazing experience."

Three months after the session, and only four months after she'd been diagnosed with her third recurrence of cancer, Marolan was in the hospital, sick from chemotherapy and an electrolyte imbalance. While she was there, the medical team performed a battery of routine tests. After viewing the results, Marolan's oncologist came into her room. He was crying, Marolan recalls, and he said, "Your cancer's gone! We don't know where it went, nobody knows where it went. But your cancer's *gone!*"

Eight years after she was first diagnosed with cancer, still suffering from debilitating pain, Marolan went to Harmony Hill for the first time.

"I think that instead of me discovering Harmony Hill, Harmony Hill kind of discovered me. I kept having the name 'fall into my hands' over and over. When I was sick, I'd think I was too sick to go, it was too far away, I was too tired to get out there, that type of thing. Then my counselor recommended it. She said, 'I think it would do you good to go.'

"I signed up for a one-day 'Living with Cancer' workshop. I was feeling strong, I could drive. I didn't need anybody else to go with me, but boy, did I need some healing. And they were there, at Harmony Hill, and they had their arms open. They cared for me in a way that I'd never been cared for before. They were absolutely selfless. Just *everything* I needed was there, and *they made me feel like I deserved to be treated that way, that I was worthy to be taken care of in a loving, nurturing way*.

"A lot of the way I'd gotten through the cancer before was 'boot-camp style.' I was sort of 'boot-camp' with myself – you know, 'Things will be just fine.' It was such a different experience for me to have people say, 'Relax, take a load off, we're here to take care of you, you know; why don't you tell us about it?'"

Marolan arrived at Harmony Hill the night before Easter Sunday, 2008. "It was a very rainy and dark day, and no one else was there yet. A woman, covered from head to toe in rain gear, met me at my car, helped carry my bags and walked me to the cottage. Standing in the doorway, Gretchen – who'd only introduced herself to me by her name, so I didn't know at the time that she was the founder – took off her hood, hugged me super-tight, and said 'I'm *so* glad that you're here.'" Marolan pauses, her voice softening at the recollection. "And I thought to myself, 'that was the most *genuine* hug I'd *ever* received in my whole life. *Ever.'*

"I had the whole place to myself that night. It was just awesome, just what I needed – time for myself, and space. And that's what I've found, every time I've gone there since that first time: The Hill gives you exactly what you need. Each experience is different, but every time, it's exactly what you need."

Today, Marolan is busy "giving back." (see Chapter 5)

"I have all these things that I want to accomplish – and my health stands between me and doing everything I want. But through lots of trial and error, I think we've finally found a good combination of pain meds; I can't tell you how blessed I feel to have even portions of the day without excruciating pain."

Marolan smiles a beatific smile. "And you know what? I believe my body's continuing to heal, to get better and better and better. I really do. I don't know why I'm staying, but I am obviously here for a reason. I don't know what it is, but I'm excited to find out." ❧

"Decide to be happy. Render others happy. Proclaim your joy. Love passionately your miraculous life...."

– DR. ROBERT MULLER

CHAPTER NINE:
Tears of transformation – navigating grief and loss

*"Being at Harmony Hill was literally a life-changing experience for me....
I feel like I overturned stones that were left untouched far too long. For the
first time in so long, I didn't feel anger over her cancer, mentally begging her
to 'buck up' and be strong. Instead, my heart finally broke. I felt pain and
sadness and empathy for her. I know why Harmony Hill is such a special
place – it has touched me in places I thought were long ago shut off.
Thank you."* – CAREGIVER WHO ATTENDED A CANCER RETREAT, 2007

Most of us grow up with the expectation that our lives will follow a more-or-less predictable path. We carry with us a vision of what life – career, marriage, family, adventures – will look like, and how we will be the hero of our own story. When life does not unfold as we expected, we may be faced with a world that feels as if it has been turned upside-down and shaken. Inevitably, there is grief for the loss of something, or someone, we had expected to be in our life. ❧

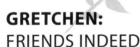

GRETCHEN:
FRIENDS INDEED

In our cancer retreats, grief is always present. Sometimes it's grief for lives cut short; sometimes it's grief for what cancer has taken away; and sometimes it's grief for our helplessness in the face of it all.

I remember a young mom who came to one of our retreats, accompanied by her dearest friend, another young mom. Emily Dade had received a terminal diagnosis; her hope was to live long enough to walk her daughter to the first day of kindergarten. She had a large circle of support – family and friends – and all were clearly grieving their impending loss. As were we at the Hill.

Harmony Hill became a place of support for Emily's family and friends both before and after her death. (She died a week short of her daughter's first day of kindergarten.) They walked the grounds. They reminisced on the bench in the arbor that looks across Hood Canal to the Olympic Mountains. They grieved, each in their own way.

I find similar comfort in the gardens at Harmony Hill. In the face of my own outrage and grief, digging in the rich soil helps me return to a space where I can be available to the people who come here.

Witnessing the outpouring of grief for Emily, and the anger and sadness of her family and friends, it became clear that a logical extension of Harmony Hill's mission would be to help people deal with grief and loss. Not just peripherally during the cancer retreats but in a retreat dedicated to this important process, a retreat where grief and loss were front and center – with all the attendant pain, anger, and regret, as well as the laughter, joy, and sweetness – for, in fact, grief contains all of these.

Thus were born Harmony Hill's grief and loss retreats. We offer them for individuals who have lost a spouse or life partner, for those who have lost a friend or family member, and, now, we've also begun developing customized programs for families to help them come together to deal with their loss in a private and very personal way.

Just like the cancer journey, the journey through grief is unique to each individual. It's neither patent nor predictable. Harmony Hill serves as a vessel to hold both grief and those grieving, and to give them a safe place to cherish their memories, express their anger, and make sense of their pain. ❧

The grief retreats at Harmony Hill follow two paths. Leonie Wolff, RNC, LMT, facilitates the retreat for those who have lost a spouse or life partner, while Linda Covert, RN, facilitates for those who have lost a loved one or family member who is not a spouse.

"We start out together, sharing our stories in circle, and we come together for meals," says Linda, "but the groups proceed in their own way, depending on the needs of the individuals present.

"Our job is to hold the space for them. We can't facilitate their healing, but we can be there for them and provide a space where they can enable their own healing."

Often healing comes in unexpected ways. Linda recalls a brother and sister who attended the Grief and Loss retreat, "Language of Loss," following the death of their beloved brother, a man in his late 40s. One of the activities attendees engaged in during the retreat was to write letters to the people they'd lost, sharing any unstated feelings or hopes, recalling special memories or unexpressed reflections. "It's like a eulogy that was never spoken," says Linda. Later, they craft letters from their loved ones to themselves, imagining what they would want to say if they had the chance.

The surviving brother found himself unable to write what he was feeling, so Linda encouraged him to go to the yurt, where art supplies are kept. Hours later, he emerged with an extraordinary collage ... and with a powerful realization. As a teenager, he had been diagnosed with cancer and had lost most of his 16th year to illness, treatment, and recovery. His young adulthood was cut short and, instead of memories of carefree teen experiences, he had carried for decades the awareness of serious illness and the fear of a shortened life. Grieving for his brother had opened up his own long-buried grief for himself.

His collage depicted a succession of activities and moods, beginning with sunny pastimes – biking and sailing – then moving to storm-darkened skies and shadowy, foreboding caves. These were followed by scenes of light and laughter.

"It just blew us all away," remembers Linda. "In the space of grieving for his brother, he was able to honor his own pain and move into it and through it. What you think you're coming here for is just the invitation. What happens here is always something more.

"We carry so much grief around with us, grief from so many losses – family members, friends, pets – not just deaths, but other losses, as well: disappointments, abandonments, dreams unfulfilled. The retreat provides a safe place to open up our souls to all of those losses. In the space of being together with others who are open to their grief, we heal, we move through it. We can't erase the sadness, but we can leave behind some of the burdens of grief. People learn how to hold the part they need to keep and allow the burden to flow through them and wash away. We keep the best parts in our heart."

In the "Passionate Sadness" retreat for grieving spouses and partners, facilitator Leonie Wolff addresses head-on the idea that all love stories end in tragedy. Calling on her own experience of holding her beloved husband in her arms as he died, Leonie strives to create a deeply nurturing environment for "those left behind."

"The death of a life partner is unique grief in that you lose the person who is the daily witness to your life. Regardless of the nature of the relationship, all aspects of *who-you-are* become deeply altered.

"Grief cannot be ignored, fought, finished, processed, analyzed or gone around. It must be gone through. We offer a safe and caring space for individuals to gather together with others who know what they are feeling when they wake up at 3:00 a.m.," says Leonie. "Over the three days of the retreat, we tell our stories and we are listened to. We explore our own wisdom. And we honor those who have left us. For a short while, we walk this difficult path together." ❧

"When one door closes another opens. But we often look so long and so regretfully upon the closed door that we fail to see the one that has opened for us."

– ALEXANDER GRAHAM BELL

JAN SIMON:
ENDURING LOVE

What Jan Simon remembers most about the Caregiver Retreat she attended in August of 2008 is the sense of freedom she felt at Harmony Hill: "It was like the load I had been carrying for so long was lifted."

For Jan, it was a brief respite not only from caring for her husband, but also from advocating for him through the medical system – fighting for insurance coverage for the stem cell transplants to treat his Hodgkin's lymphoma, fighting for care from doctors and nurses in a system that doesn't always put the patient first.

"He was lucky to have a bossy wife," she says with a smile. "But it was hard to stop fighting, or to slow down."

That sort of advocacy is exhausting, especially in a treatment regimen that requires sometimes daily hospital visits, as well as extreme care with meals and the home environment for a patient whose immune system has been totally suppressed to accommodate the transplant. "At Harmony Hill all of that was lifted from me, and even after, it didn't come back in the same way.

"The experience of being looked in the eyes, and listened to, and being with people who understand what you're going through ... it doesn't leave you the same."

Nothing more perfectly describes for Jan her experience at Harmony Hill than the Meister Eckhart poem, "Love Does That."

LOVE DOES THAT
All day long a little burro labors, sometimes
with heavy loads on her back and sometimes just with worries
about things that bother only
burros.
And worries, as we know, can be more exhausting
than physical labor.
Once in a while a kind monk comes
to her stable and brings
a pear, but more
than that,
he looks into the burro's eyes and touches her ears
and for a few seconds the burro is free
and even seems to laugh,
because love does
that.
Love Frees.

Jan recalls a powerful question that was posed to caregivers during the retreat: *How far will you go?*

"Until that moment, I never saw the path I was on as a choice, but it was. Accompanying Alain was my choice. We all had a choice in our roles as caregivers, and I could choose *how far I would go*. Being able to examine what I was going through as if it was a choice – as if I had a say in the matter – changed the way I saw the journey. It had never occurred to me not to do it, and I never would have considered not accompanying him every step of the way, but, somehow, seeing it as a choice changed the way I felt about it. It was empowering and also liberating."

Alain died four months later, and Jan continued alone down the corridor of grief she and her husband had embarked upon when his doctor told them the transplant and subsequent chemotherapy had not been successful. In some ways, Jan says, their journey together through cancer was almost a gift.

"His treatment was brutal, but he did it with so much grace, and humor, and love. Alain and I went through something that was so intimate. It was such a privilege to go through that with him. It was real, immediate, authentic, and it was precious. It's life writ large. We used to joke: we haven't walked through the valley of the shadow of death, we set up camp there. You don't go on a journey like that and come out the same."

Describing how the journey changed her, Jan says, "I'm a nicer person. I have a tenderness and vulnerability that I'm not afraid of showing. I like people more, too. And I like myself more...I like life more. I see that there's more to life. I still worry about the little things, but I see there's more."

Jan attended the "Passionate Sadness" Grief Retreat at Harmony Hill about nine months after her husband's death. Again, she experienced the gift of listening and being listened to.

"Going there, I felt like I had to be with others of my species, other people who *know*. We were all part of a tribe we didn't want to be a part of. We shared so much with one another. Some people had regrets they needed to speak of. Many talked of the courage their spouse or partner had shown. We talked about how they faced their death with such heart and such dignity. Being able to honor that among people who really understand – that was incredible."

To others dealing with grief, Jan offers, "Be nice to yourself. No matter what, be good to yourself. Accept however you are. Know that you're on a roller coaster. Life will sneak up on you.

"Each person's grief is theirs alone. People don't know how to be with you. And

> "If the doors of perception were cleansed, everything would appear to man as it is – infinite. For man has closed himself up, till he sees all things through narrow chinks of his cavern."
>
> – WILLIAM BLAKE

just because I've been through it, I don't know either. The important thing is just to be there, to offer what you can. It doesn't have to be perfect. It just has to be."

Jan purchased one of the paving bricks in Harmony Hill's tribute path and had it inscribed in memory of her beloved husband.

"I've been back to Harmony Hill a few times since, and the first thing I do when I get there is go to it. I touch it, I talk to him ... it's almost like he's there waiting for me. It's comforting," Jan says, *"to know it will always be there."* ❧

DANETTE KELLY-COSTELLO:
HEEDING THE CALL

Danette Kelly-Costello was in the midst of a personal crisis when she arrived at Harmony Hill in 1997 for a three-day personal retreat. Meeting Gretchen for the first time, Danette said hello then collapsed into Gretchen's arms, weeping. The next thing she said was, "I promise you I'm going to recover from this and I'm going to come back out here and help you."

Fourteen years later, Danette is still making good on her promise.

Danette grew up in Hawaii. When she was eight years old, she witnessed a healer doing bodywork on her mother's back and had a profound spiritual experience.

"This man was listening to something clear as my voice, seeing something clear as a cup of tea before me. As I watched him, somehow I understood *that I am, as I was and always will be, something you can never put in a bottle.* Shortly after that, when I was in school, our class was assigned to write about what we wanted to be when we grow up. As I was writing, I heard the *click, click, click* of my teacher's heels as she walked around the room, surveying the students at work. When the clicking stopped behind me, I knew she was reading over my shoulder, looking at my answer. I'd written 'spiritual healer.' The teacher asked, 'Do you mean a nurse?' *Oh, dear,* I realized, *I'm not supposed to share this....*"

She never wavered, however, in pursuit of her calling. When she was nineteen, she trained with the great Lomi Lomi teacher, Kahuna (healer) Aunty Margaret Machado. Aunty Margaret was a living legend in Hawaii. Besides learning massage, there was much hard work involved in the apprenticeship. Danette, like all the apprentices, started at the very bottom, which meant doing the least glamorous tasks one might imagine, such as emptying the intestinal-cleansing buckets.

She stuck with and completed the training, and eventually left Hawaii, feeling as if she was "leaving the mythological garden behind" as she moved into the rest of the world. When she settled in the community of Poulsbo, Washington, Danette began working with cancer patients and people with past injuries. She continues her healing massage practice today.

Over the years since Danette's introduction to the Hill, she would visit from time to time – renting the yurt and taking groups of people out there to do spiritual work. She has facilitated healing meditations and singing for cancer retreat participants. It was Danette's very first visit, however, that really set the stage for the work in which she's been most recently involved – a Grief and Loss retreat.

Grappling with a personal crisis, including a struggle with Lyme disease, Danette's first Harmony Hill stay was in the cottage. The woman who was living in the cottage at the time wasn't there, but her Siamese cat was. Once she'd settled in, Danette filled the big claw-foot tub with warm water and sank into it. The tub, filled to overflow, was noisily trickling into the drain, and the cat began to yowl like only a Siamese can.

"I thought, 'What on earth is going on here?' Because I was at Harmony Hill, where I could allow myself the time to just be, I lay there until I realized that I hadn't dealt with grief."

The moment she had this epiphany, two things happened: the water stopped, and the cat curled up and went to sleep.

"I'd gotten to a place where I was safe to deal with the grief. There was so much emotional pressure built up inside, and I'd been too busy 'outside' to pay attention," Danette reflects. "If we don't attend our inner world, our outer world will mirror what we must tend. I'd been walking around with screaming cats inside!

"When you're in that place of separation, a Harmony Hill retreat gives you the chance to recalibrate, to come alive, to reconnect your inner and outer world. And you don't have to receive the teaching in a linear way. If you're open, like a quartz radio, things will pop into your head.

"There's a profound resonance, so hard to put into words, at Harmony Hill; the place has an energetic integrity. When I'm there, I don't want to disturb a single thing...."

Danette was one of the faculty for the first private Grief and Loss retreat held at Harmony Hill in 2010 – the prototype for a program aimed to help people cope with grief and loss of all kinds, not just those dealing with cancer.

"The Grief and Loss retreat was life-changing for me. Meeting facilitators J Fields and Lu Farber was a profound experience. And a particular moment of the family's retreat really stands out for me: One family member showed up, saying that this wasn't really her thing, she'd rather be hiking. She scheduled a massage with me because... well, everyone has their own way of dealing with grief. I was playing classical Debussy and the sunlight was hitting the beautiful autumn leaves, the wind blowing. And I thought, hey, we're having a spiritual moment here despite ourselves, aren't we? The man for whom the family was grieving was present in everything around us, joined back into the force of life – the sun and the leaves. You know, when we shut ourselves within our house, in our bodies, we can't open that door; we never feel comfortable with that part of our body, where we've denied it.

"Years ago, when I was considering doing hospice work, I looked up the definition for hospice. We tend to think of it as a place for the dying, but its first definition is 'to give shelter and refuge to pilgrims on their journey, sanctuary when it's hard.'

"And that is what Harmony Hill provides: shelter and refuge to pilgrims on their journey, sanctuary when it's hard. That is its purpose. *Harmony Hill is a divine hospital – you may not find a cure there, but you are going to receive healing."* ❧

> " The friend who can be silent with us in a moment of despair or confusion, who can stay with us in an hour of grief and bereavement,   who can tolerate not knowing... not healing, not curing... that is a friend who cares."
>
> – HENRI NOUWEN

HELEN RAIKES AND FAMILY:
GRIEVING TOGETHER AND HEALING TOGETHER

Ron Raikes was 66 years old when he was killed in a tractor accident on his family farm in Nebraska. The accident occurred on Labor Day in 2009. A well-respected former state senator acknowledged for his leadership in the field of education, Ron was known far and wide for his intelligence, integrity, and wry humor. He was also a farmer, educator, father and husband. His death shocked and saddened a wide community of friends and family.

Many months later, as the anniversary of Ron's death approached, his wife Helen felt a need to find something to mark the occasion – to honor Ron's memory and to help the family members who were each dealing with their grief and loss in their own way.

"I knew I at least had a need to do something focused to remember Ron in a special way on that day," says Helen Raikes, Willa Cather Professor of Child, Youth and Family Studies at the University of Nebraska-Lincoln, and also a consultant to the U.S. Department of Health and Human Services. "I also knew I wanted to be with family."

Helen talked to her sister-in-law and, along with one of Helen's daughters, they hatched an idea to offer a "grief retreat" for the family, and to offer it at Harmony Hill. The family has a home nearby and was familiar with the Hill.

"When the suggestion first came up," Helen continues, "My response was, 'I don't think so...this is too much. I've been processing my grief every day and I don't know if I can do this or even want to do this.' I worried that if we all came together for something this intense I might not be strong enough to take care of everybody and hold the weight of their grief. I knew we were all at different stages of grieving. Some hadn't processed it much; some had done a lot of processing. Everyone would be responding differently.

"It was good for me to get in touch with that and to realize that it would be okay to say to everybody, 'We're all on our own … we're all together, but we're each going to take our own path.' That was okay.

"Also, I couldn't picture my son participating in something like this. He was dealing with his grief privately, and this was just so – *public*. I knew what Ron would have said about it. He'd have called it a 'group grope' and walked out the door within five minutes. Our son might feel the same way as his dad about something of this nature.

"We talked about it more. What was proposed was too structured. We talked with Gretchen and the facilitators about what we felt we needed and what we envisioned. We needed to build in space for each of us to work through our own issues. We needed to offer 'escape hatches' for any activities that anyone might be uncomfortable with. Even though it was a group experience, everyone needed to be able to choose to be in or out at any time. Together, we crafted a plan that was both structured and fluid, with plenty of open space.

"As we were planning it I called my son and described to him what we had in mind. His response to me was courteous, 'Oh, that's nice,' he said, but just moments later his sister got a text message from him saying *'WTF.'*" Helen laughs. "He was being so kind, but it clearly didn't sound to him like something he would be keen on."

As it turned out, though, her son – and the other men of the family who Helen thought might be skeptical – came to the retreat and participated in just about everything.

"It offered choices. We could do yoga, or not. We could journal, or go for a walk. The guys stayed with it all the way. We all saw that the whole weekend was about us coming together over Ron. It was okay if someone just wanted to come and hang out. We all had permission to deal with our grief in whatever way worked for us."

Helen tried not to have many expectations for the weekend. But whatever expectations she had or didn't have were exceeded.

"I certainly didn't go into it with any expectation that I would be in a different place afterwards."

But things did change for her: "For me, something shifted after that weekend. I have enough respect for the grief process to know not to try to drive it, but to let it take the course it needs to take. I just listen and try to respond. I had been very sad – not overtly depressed – but deeply sad. My wish after months of sadness was to be able to experience joy again, to not continually be coming back to grief, to feel engaged again. And I think that shift happened for me within that circle of caring.

"I came away from Harmony Hill feeling different. I *am* more engaged. I am more productive. I laugh more. I still miss Ron terribly, but the searing pain has softened."

Ten members of Helen's family attended the retreat. The first day was just for Helen and her two daughters, one of whom had an obligation that prevented her from staying for the whole weekend. During that day they shared memories of Ron and of their life with him. After that, they did a long restorative yoga session together. Then they shared some more.

"Talking and yoga – the three of us were very comfortable with those modalities," says Helen.

On the second day, more family members joined them. Each had a massage and Helen recalls that the massage therapist later said "she felt she knew our family story through our bodies after the fourth or fifth person."

The moment during the retreat that took Helen's breath away was during her own massage. Before the treatment started, she warned Danette that at different times she had broken a leg and a wrist and both were still somewhat cranky.

"Then while she was massaging near my chest, I started sobbing and sobbing and couldn't stop. When it was over, I told her, 'Oh, I forgot to tell you about my broken heart.' 'Yes,' she said, 'yes, but I found it.'"

On day three, the family spent a lot more time sharing. They talked about Ron's legacy; they talked about what he would have been proud of; they shared regrets and treasured memories. Ron had been known for his tremendous sense of humor, and they remembered hilarious things he had said or speculated on the comical comments he would have made had he been with them. Each person shared one special thing that he or she wanted to remember about Ron.

"There were a lot of tears and a lot of laughter," recalls Helen.

Throughout the retreat they also had opportunities to journal, walk the labyrinth, and to write a letter to Ron recalling any special memories or stating anything that may have been left unsaid. They were free to share or to keep private their reflections. Ron's nephew, Connor, wrote a poem that conveyed the depth of his loss and his deep regard for his uncle. When he shared it, it touched the family deeply.

The Fallen Tree
by Connor Raikes

I look upon a newly fallen tree
A'taken in the cruel unruly night
It ne'er before impressed itself on me
And only now I see its silent might

For once it stood unwavering and stout
Alone upon a hill; a beacon high
The thick and tested branches reaching out
And holding up what bird would come on by

Through wind and rain it stood through great tumult
The tangled roots ne'er straying from the earth
It fell at last unto a lightning bolt
The rot to feed and hold new seeds to birth

Since on't I could so easily depend
I failed to see (forgive me!) till the end.

(Dedicated to Ron Raikes)

Although some of the retreat work was done at the family home near Harmony Hill, Helen credits much of the success of the retreat to the beauty of the setting: "It couldn't have been any more ideal. The view of the Hood Canal and the Olympic Mountains is magnificent. And there is a sense of sacredness there – both in the physical nature of the place and in the approach the facilitators take to everything they do. The facilitators who worked with us were so respectful; they watched and listened, and took their cues from us. A retreat like this brings up intense feelings - our retreat was a safe container for those feelings and for all that energy. We relaxed together in the midst of that healing energy.

> **"Your pain is the breaking of the shell that encloses your understanding."**
>
> – KHALIL GIBRAN

"For me," Helen says, "having the physicality of the yoga and the massage, together with the sharing and the personal reflection – it was a powerful three-way approach to healing. I can't speak for other members of our family, but it felt like everyone experienced a shift of some kind. It feels like we are all more able to be engaged in the world again."

Remarking on the experience of profound grief and loss, Helen notes that "even grief presents opportunities for the resiliency and creativity of the human spirit to emerge. It's inspiring to see how people approach grief out of their own needs and their own creativity, how they find ways to heal and move forward. Having a retreat was our way to do it.

"People often create community around loss. In the midst of profound pain there are authentic feelings to be honored and creative moments to be shared – and out of these there can be healing.

"For anybody who might be contemplating something like this, know that it brings up some pretty intense feelings, not just about the grief, but about how you want to process it. But out of all that, healing can happen." ❖

PATTY MULHERN, RN, MN:
FRIEND AND MENTOR

Each of the VOICE nurses will tell you that Patty Mulhern was the driving force behind their community. Patty had been a housemom at Harmony Hill for many years and when these seven women connected to advance their vision to promote healing for health professionals, Patty was the glue that sustained that connection. Patty died in 2009 after her own struggle with cancer. She had recently retired from a 30-plus-year career in home health care.

"This was where Patty envisioned her future. She had made the shift professionally and created the space to focus on renewal for nurses and other health care professionals," says her VOICE colleague Kathlene Tellgren.

When Patty turned 60, she asked her VOICE sisters to help her acknowledge that transition. She asked Kathlene to facilitate a "croning ceremony" at Harmony Hill.

"I didn't even know what that was," recalls Kathlene. "I had to Google it. But what we put together was a beautiful ritual acknowledging Patty's first 60 years and her entrance into the next part of her journey. We set candles around the perimeter of the labyrinth and Patty walked it alone. It was a crisp, autumn evening and the moon and stars were shining brightly. When we greeted her as she walked out of the labyrinth, we were welcoming and embracing the wise woman who had, both literally and figuratively, stepped into her wisdom."

That ceremony – a public declaration of her wisdom – marked a transition for Patty. It became ever so clear to her that VOICE was her next step. She recognized and accepted that her mission and purpose was to embody the voice for healers and share that piece of herself.

Over the next months, Patty worked on developing Harmony Hill's programs for health professionals, and she joined Gretchen and Kathlene on the Scottish island of Iona, where together they facilitated a week-long retreat for health professionals in transition. Patty also continued her career-long practice of mentoring other nurses.

Fellow VOICE nurse Rosemary Spyhalsky, RN, OCN, HN-BC, was one of the nurses Patty mentored. As the youngest of the group, Rosemary first came to Harmony Hill at a time of personal crisis.

"I felt separated from my heart and spirit, separated even from the wholeness of the patients I was seeing as a chemo and oncology nurse. Harmony Hill was where I saw that there was another way to be as a nurse, and where I came to understand the concept of holistic nursing.

"Patty became a mentor to me as I started in my current position as Nurse Coordinator of the Integrative Care program. She was always there to offer her advice and experience, and, most of all, her encouragement. It was so very valuable to me to know that I could call Patty – and I did, multiple times – and each and every time she would be there for me, a wise and caring advisor to whom I could talk about the subtle nuances of a situation. An administrative role was new to me, and Patty gently guided me through some of my crucial first steps. I have missed her so much. Many times, in various work settings, I have found myself thinking: *I wish I could call Patty right now... I wonder what Patty would say.*"

When Patty Mulhern died at age 62, the group faltered somewhat. Recalls Linda Covert, "We were like a circle that had lost its center."

Now, though, the collective grief for Patty has taken many forms and opened some new doors for the group and for Harmony Hill.

"Patty's death moved us to finding our own individual voices out of our collective voice," notes Kathlene Tellgren.

Linda adds, "I have come to embrace more closely the voice that I use on a daily basis. My intention each day when I walk into that building is to mentor, encourage, and support nurses and nursing through my words and my work."

The "Embracing" program is moving ahead – in both one-day and three-day formats. Nurse renewal has become a major parallel focus of Harmony Hill. There are connections and partnerships with the American Holistic Nurses Association and NIGH, the Nightingale Initiative on Global Health, a grassroots, nurse-inspired movement to increase awareness about health as a global, public priority, and to empower nurses and concerned citizens to lead the way.

Increasingly, health care organizations are sending nurses to Harmony Hill to participate in the renewal programs, or inviting the Hill to replicate the programs at their facilities. Harmony Hill is on the path to becoming the Northwest Center for Nurse Renewal. The VOICE nurses, with Patty Mulhern at their center, formed the foundation from which these exciting opportunities are evolving.

"Patty's spirit shows up here often," says Gretchen.

"Patty was a connector. Part of her legacy is the expansion of the vision for nursing renewal to administrative levels within healthcare systems and into academia. We had a vision of being instrumental in changing healthcare, and it's happening – one nurse at a time, one heart at a time." ❧

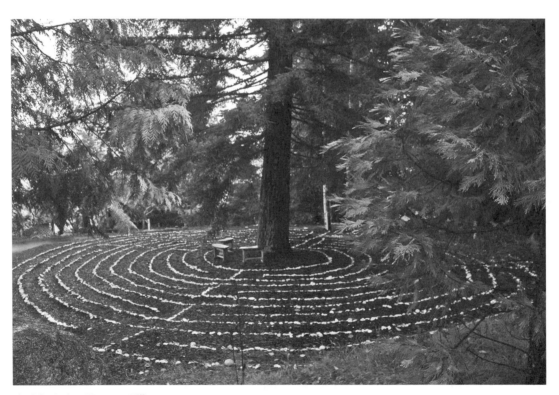

The labyrinth at Harmony Hill.

CHAPTER TEN:
Homecoming

"I came here knowing I had locked something up inside myself....
This experience has enabled me to unlock the door and see for the first
time in a long time." – EMILY DADE, 2003

Some people who visit Harmony Hill find it hard to describe the feeling they had the first time they saw the Hill. Some have called it an "enchantment" – an infusion of wonder and oneness, a sense of magic and dreamlike possibilities. Others express it as a sense of wholeness – a union of body, mind, and spirit that offers a newfound sense of clarity. Perhaps the word most frequently used to describe the feeling of coming to Harmony Hill – whether for the first time or the fiftieth – is "homecoming." ❖

JO WHITACRE:
A CARING TEAM MEMBER

Jo Whitacre is a key member of Harmony Hill's hospitality staff. She found Harmony Hill at a time when she needed support. Not only did she find the sustenance she needed, she became a pillar of the caring team that supports so many individuals each year – with love, compassion, and individual attention.

Jo recalls the challenges she was facing in 2000: "That year, my beautiful parents passed away, and I went through a divorce. For renewal and healing, I looked outward to find a change from some difficult Tacoma memories. A year later, on the Hood Canal in Union, I found *two* new homes – one to live in, and the other was Harmony Hill."

Jo volunteered at the Hill for about six months and then was offered a hospitality position.

"It's given me a new family, much laughter, a few tears, and abundant rewards, thanks to our mission, our caring staff, and our retreat participants.

"As a hospitality staff member," Jo notes, "my nurturing side, my teacher side, and my make-the-place-look-inviting side are all fed. Preparing the buildings for retreats, making flower arrangements, building welcoming fires, greeting retreatants, and giving orientations and labyrinth talks all allow me to do what I love. Often, I get to shuttle participants to and from Harmony Hill in our van. This is when I really get to know them, hear their stories, learn about their anxieties at facing a cancer retreat, or revel with them at their first glimpse of Hood Canal and the Olympic Mountains. I remember one cancer retreat participant who was overcome with joy and tears when she was greeted by mile after mile of wildly colorful springtime azaleas and rhodies all along Highway 106."

Jo finds it exhilarating to experience the collective energy of the myriad groups that come to Harmony Hill.

"There are the business group meetings which, while mostly business, always make time to enjoy their surroundings. The Nonviolent Communicators are very playful and such caring listeners. The Mystery School gives off a loving, mysterious glow. The nursing and hospice groups nurture us all to no end. The cancer retreats are the most inspiring, emotion-filled groups. These participants are so brave, and they give so much back without realizing it, adding to the amazing vibrancy of this space. Then, there are the weddings, the celebrations, the music...such joy filling the Hill!"

Jo recently experienced being a participant in one of the Hill's programs.

"Tai Ji Master Chungliang Al Huang led a powerful and joyful three-day seminar which opened me up much more in the realm of giving and receiving energy. I will take this practice into my daily life, especially into my work. Because I was a three-day participant, I now know first-hand how our retreat participants experience our offerings. The Great Hall is truly a magnificent space! And the hospitality and food are exceptional, just as we so often hear. When several of my fellow participants heard that I work here, they were envious and quick to ask how they might work here, too. We made sure they were given volunteer forms; we just might see them again, and again."

"I am thankful and very proud to be a part of the Harmony Hill family. The Hill was here for me when I was in need of nurturing. I will continue to give back as I can." ❖

GRETCHEN:
NO PLACE LIKE HOME...

Harmony Hill has now been my home for 25 years. For the first eight years, I lived in the lodge, first in a tiny bedroom that is now across from our gift nook, then in a larger room that served half as bedroom and half as office. My barracks were close to the kitchen, where, in the early years, I was chief cook and bottle-washer.

As we refocused our mission on offering cancer programs, it became clear that I needed to make some changes, too. It was hard for me to give up my work in the kitchen – for me, cooking is deeply pleasurable, as well as the best kind of therapy (matched only by gardening!) Cindy Shank had joined the staff by then, and she was willing and able to take on more responsibilities in the kitchen. As we grew, we added permanent kitchen staff. I am continually amazed by the wizardry and dedication of our kitchen crew. It's evident that our guests feel the same way. Many returnees have told us that they came back for the food!

At the same time that I disengaged from the kitchen, I moved out of the lodge and into the newly-jacked-up cabin. Despite occasional structural challenges – such as when the floor under my bed caved in – it was a rustic, but cozy, setting for my quarters and office. I stayed there for a few years and then moved into a trailer next door. From its porch, I enjoyed glorious views of sunsets over the Hood Canal; it was easy to pretend I was living on a sailboat. This perfect location later became the site of the Creekside building. People who stay in the rooms there still remark on the breathtaking views.

In 2001, I moved to the new apartment in the upper level of the facilities building. It felt like I was moving into a castle – still does! This was our first Built Green™ building and such a comfort to come home to after I was diagnosed with non-Hodgkin's lymphoma. ❖

J FIELDS:
THE LESSONS OF CANCER

J Fields has been facilitating cancer retreats at Harmony Hill since 2004. His path to the Hill followed his own cancer experience in 2003. Diagnosed with bladder cancer, which was later discovered to have metastasized, he endured grueling treatment, including complications with chemo that brought him to the brink.

"Throughout treatment, I kept a gratefulness journal, listing five things each day that I was grateful for. Sometimes number one was just that I wasn't throwing up. Chemo was tough!"

J was also grateful for, and even a bit surprised by how much support he had from friends and family.

"It helped me through. When I was diagnosed, so many friends came forward to help me; my daughters were there for me every step of the way. One friend even used his entire two weeks of vacation to come and care for me. That was the first lesson cancer taught me: that I was lovable. That's a powerful lesson, and it made me want to keep going."

There were other lessons, as well: "Cancer changed my life totally. I remember lying in bed and seeing the drops of rain in the branches and the sun shining through, and thinking how beautiful life is, how precious – and how temporary. And I thought about how I wanted to spend my energy. I took a medical retirement from my job. While I won't call cancer a gift, the lessons it gave me changed my life, and I knew I wanted to give back."

Melissa West introduced J to Harmony Hill. He went out to the Hill thinking he was interviewing to be a volunteer, but they invited him to join the faculty as the first male facilitator for cancer retreats. His background in therapy and counseling and his own journey through cancer have equipped him with the skills and perspective to connect deeply with retreat participants.

"As a facilitator, I need to know when to step in to guide the group, and when to step back and allow the group to go where it needs to go with its own internal and collective leadership."

Today, J leads about six three-day retreats each year, and he coordinates the faculty at Harmony Hill.

"Every group that comes out here is different, and no retreat is the same as any other. For me, cancer was an incredibly transformative experience, and I want to help people have an experience that is transformative for them. But you can't teach healing – our job is to provide the space, and some tools, to help people make their choices and get in touch with their own healing."

There can be healing without cure, and sometimes cure without healing. J recalls a recent retreat, unusual in the fact that five of the participants were men – there are usually fewer. Patrick was one of the attendees.

"He was a biker, a big guy, tattooed, wearing leathers, the kind of guy you give some space to walking down the street. When we opened the retreat in circle to share our stories, Patrick asked to go first. He said if he didn't he was afraid he wouldn't be able to. He described his experience with cancer a few years earlier. For him, it had been a lonely time and he had felt completely isolated; he recalled coming home from chemo and being completely alone. He still carried the scars of that loneliness and pain. As he described the pain of that isolation, he began to cry. His crying – *his being able to cry* – opened up the room for everybody else. It was such a powerful moment and we were all in awe of his courage and his openness. Even though Patrick was cancer-free at the time he attended the retreat, *that* moment was really when his healing began."

J likens the trauma of an initial cancer diagnosis to the horror of 9/11.

"Suddenly you feel that your life is no longer safe. Your world has changed. It's like being dropped into the jungle without a map or having your life swept away by a tornado. You go from this shock and chaos to a survival mode where you're making hard choices and decisions about treatment. Then, there's a place beyond the fear where you find some new meaning – either in the cancer or in your life, and eventually you come to your own peace."

J says he learns much from each group he works with, and from every participant.

"I see a person with a terminal diagnosis who says just the right thing to help another person. I see the tenderness between a husband and wife that is such pure love it takes your breath away. I see a level of honesty that allows people to say what is really there – sometimes for the first time ever. They can admit that they're lost or terrified, or they can ask for help, and, among strangers, they are accepted – *totally accepted* – just as they are."

Asked to explain the magic, J points to the grounds: "It's this place, its physical beauty; it's also Gretchen's vision unfolding, and it's the staff, and the faculty, and the housemoms. We all have the same purpose: to provide a safe place for people to find healing. That's our mission here at Harmony Hill."

The magic of Harmony Hill isn't evident only to retreat participants. J feels it every time he drives up the driveway.

"It feels like I'm coming home. It's a place of belonging. There's something about the land – it feels special. It feels sacred, and you can feel the energy of all the people who work here and who have come here."

When asked how he describes Harmony Hill to others, J just says, "Oh, you gotta come!" Then he adds, "This is a place for healing. This is a place for you to come and just be you. A lot of cancer patients feel isolated; sometimes friends disappear, sometimes you are alone. Here's a place you can come to and share who you are, warts and all. It's a safe space to be completely real and discover whatever it is that you need to do for yourself." ❖

> **"Learn to be quiet enough to hear the genuine within yourself so that you can hear it in others."**
>
> – MARIAN WRIGHT EDELMAN

CINDY SHANK:
AN OPEN PASSION

Some lucky folks like their jobs, but how often do you hear someone say, "My work has transformed every aspect of my life"? That's how Harmony Hill's Program Manager Cindy Shank describes hers.

Cindy first discovered Harmony Hill in August 1995, when she attended the Wellness Festival with her two daughters and her aunt.

"During that event, I fell in love with the natural beauty and energy of the Hill, and then shortly after the festival I saw an ad in the local paper for a household/kitchen assistant."

Though she'd worked before her children were born, Cindy had been out of the working world for many years. In her mind, Cindy saw a circle of women doing good work together in that beautiful place, and she wanted to be part of that circle. She wrote a letter to Gretchen, who called Cindy for an interview, and by early September, Cindy was on staff part-time as a kitchen/household assistant.

At that time, the staff was very small, and Cindy's job included everything from supervising work crews from the women's correctional center to cleaning out the basement. Eventually, she became the Accommodations Coordinator, a role in which she supervised staff, planned menus and cooked meals for groups and programs for the first five years. She then moved into the role of Cancer Program Assistant, then Coordinator, then Program Manager.

As Program Manager, Cindy oversees the program lineup; she develops new programs and refines and manages existing ones. She's responsible for hiring, orienting and managing the faculty for the cancer and wellness programs, for handling all wellness program registrations and details, and she is also a member of the Leadership Team.

She's learned a lot about change during her years at Harmony Hill, noting that "most change is good, although it's not always apparent when you're in the midst of it. We've been through some tough times over the years, but in the end, they created growth and opportunities that never could have been imagined.

"I've seen so many miracles happen here: volunteers showing up, seemingly out of nowhere, when we were in a major staff shortage; financial support coming right when we need it the most to keep us going through tight spots, and, of course, the incredible transformations of those who have attended our cancer program.

"So many times I greet participants on the first day of a cancer retreat, often finding them withdrawn, scared and almost angry to be in this place where they feel so vulnerable. By the last day of the retreat, these people are transformed. They're laughing, crying (good tears), and often not wanting to leave the sacred community they have become part of – a place where they feel unconditionally loved and accepted.

"Of course, they do leave and re-enter their lives, having found what they needed to help them heal and to move forward with hope and newfound faith in their ability to cope with whatever challenges they face ahead."

Transformation is a two-way street, as Cindy found at one of the first cancer retreats in which she was involved. She was busy in the kitchen, preparing lunch for the retreat participants, when a new attendee arrived.

Their eyes met, and Cindy felt an immediate soul connection to the woman, whose name was Marion.

"She was a gracious lady in her 70s and had advanced ovarian cancer. Marion became a spiritual inspiration to me, and during the rest of her cancer journey we were special friends. She supported me during a very difficult divorce and personal crisis. I supported her however I could during her last days. She had lost most of her ability to digest food, so taking a small bite of something tasty was a huge blessing for her. Marion helped me remember what was important, to value the simple things in life – like how wonderful a small bite of cookie could taste....I was so blessed to have known her."

During the course of her work in the caring community of Harmony Hill, Cindy has met her best friends and also her husband, Gregg, whom she married in 2000 on the grounds of Harmony Hill.

"Working at the Hill has opened me up to so many wonderful people and experiences. I feel connected to a community that has consistently evolved and grown over the sixteen years I've been here. The support from my coworkers and mentors over the years has made it possible for me to open myself up to an array of creative outlets. I've grown professionally and personally, and achieved goals that I never would have thought possible.

"One of my favorite things in the world is to design space, and I've been given some wonderful opportunities to express my passion in many ways at Harmony Hill. Recently I had the privilege of decorating several new guest rooms (in the recently-constructed Gatehouse), and I enjoyed every minute of it!

"I'm invested in the work we do," Cindy says, "I am a regular donor, and contribute a small part of each paycheck back to the Hill....I like knowing that I'm helping in my own small way, personally, to help us continue that work." ❖

> **"**There is a way to live that makes the angels cry out in rapture. There is a way to live that makes each cell a star."
>
> – MORGAN FARLEY

GRETCHEN:
HOME, HEARTH, AND HEART

There's no question that the magic of this place contributes to the sense of homecoming so many people feel when they arrive at Harmony Hill – whether for the first time or the hundredth. And it's also the magic of these people – the amazing team of individuals who work here – that creates that feeling of arriving at where you belong, where you are welcome without hesitation and accepted without judgment.

One of Harmony Hill's core values is "nurturing hospitality," stated as: *We believe hospitality is at the heart of our mission – welcoming all of our guests with gratitude, and feeding and nurturing each individual.* We take that value and those words very seriously. But sometimes, taking something seriously means taking it lightly.

Mary Liz Chaffee was a member of our earliest hospitality team. Among her many responsibilities was the coordination of house-moms. She was infamous for the wild and wacky hats and earrings she often wore. They were colorful, seasonal, fun, and always something to look forward to. "What will Mary Liz's hat be today?" we'd wonder, and we were never disappointed! It became one of my joys to be on the lookout for a new hat for Mary Liz.

At Thanksgiving, Mary Liz's head was adorned with a good-sized turkey atop a plate of vegetables. In December, she treated us to an "advent calendar" of hats – starting on December 1 and becoming progressively more outrageous up until Christmas Day.

For our cancer retreat participants as well as Hill staff, Mary Liz's hats were a wonderful reminder to appreciate the absurd and invite surprise into our lives. One woman who had lost her hair to chemo told us around the closing circle that she couldn't wait to go hat shopping when she got back home. It was time to replace her bandanas with a bolder fashion statement. "I want people to look at my head and smile, not pity me," she said. She later sent us a photo of herself wearing a hat that looked like a spring garden – complete with birds *and* bees! The smile on her face said it all.

While zany hats may not be the choice for others on our staff, each and every one of our team embodies hospitality in everything they do – from making beds, to cooking nutritious meals, pruning rose bushes, or answering the phone.

Whether it's a cozy fire in the fireplace, vases of flowers everywhere, a soothing cup of tea, a hug, a smile, or just the right word, we are passionate about welcoming every guest into our "home," and making them feel as if they are the most important person in the world.

So many people have commented on the magic continually conjured by our kitchen staff that I am probably being redundant, but I still marvel at what our chefs and cooking staff do every day with such grace. They have become expert in dealing with special dietary concerns and mindfully preparing meals customized to the needs of guests. It is *never* an imposition to prepare a meal for someone with special needs. They delight not only in the preparation but also in the presentation. They create little cards to accompany those special dishes on the buffet table; the cards artfully display the guest's name and describe the dish. Recently a guest was moved to tears by the abundance of delicious gluten-free choices she was able to enjoy during a retreat – "none tasting like cardboard!" she raved.

Among the countless creative and delicious dishes prepared at the Hill, several are consistently named as favorites by our guests, among them: golden lasagna (made with yams and hazelnuts), broccoli enchiladas, Hungarian mushroom soup, spinach spanakopita, carrot cake, and practically anything we serve with fresh, local blueberries! In response to so many requests for recipes, we've published the *Harmony Hill Cookbook*, now in its fourth edition.

Food should be a joy, and sharing food together is one of the deep pleasures of being human. I'm proud that Harmony Hill's hospitality is such a visible and celebrated part of our story. ❖

LU AND STU FARBER:
LOVE AND FAMILY

Lu and Stu Farber have many reasons to celebrate the vision and gifts of Harmony Hill. The Farbers have been part of Harmony Hill's extended family since 1999. They've contributed a great deal in helping to guide the organization, they've celebrated many happy occasions on the Hill, and they've both found great comfort and support in the community during their personal bouts with cancer.

Stu was the medical director at Hospice of Tacoma when he was invited to be on the newly-formed medical advisory board in 1999.

"The idea was presented; it sounded very forward-thinking, and I think I just said yes, though I hadn't been out there yet."

What brought Lu to Harmony Hill was the labyrinth.

"I had just completed my training to be a hospice volunteer, and we had used the labyrinth extensively in that work for self-reflection. I was quite enamored of it as a tool, and had been told that Harmony Hill had one. I knew nothing at all of Harmony Hill at that point."

To celebrate her 50th birthday, she and a friend went to Harmony Hill to walk the labyrinth.

"We were doing this wonderful smudging ritual when Gretchen came up and said, essentially, 'Who are you and what are you doing here?' – in a very nice way, of course. She invited us to have tea. It was only then that I realized that Stu had been invited to be on their health advisory board. I hadn't made the connection until that very moment!"

The couple went out together for Stu's first visit to the Hill in March of '99. Stu was impressed with Gretchen and her vision and the beauty of the spot. He knew of the Commonweal program and its underlying philosophy, and was excited about having that kind of program in the area.

"Peripherally, I am very supportive," he says. "Lu's been much more involved in the day-to-day operations than I have."

Lu interjects: "Stu has a very creative mind and a good ability, particularly, to look at situations around wellness and health care, and to offer some really good insights. Gretchen admires his ability, as do I, to offer unique perspectives that have a lot of value.

"For my part," she continues, "it's been an interesting growth and development process for both Harmony Hill and me. There were some similarities and synergy to what we were going through. When I started at Harmony Hill, it was still very much in its infancy.

"I was on the board for seven years. During that time, I think I was able to add value because my background is working with organizations in significant change (in investments and in business), the strategic side of that planning. Susan Keith came on shortly after I did, and I think we made a pretty darn good team because she brought complementary skills to mine; we got some much-needed structure into place. With a lot of heartache and laughter and tears, and with the help of a lot of good and right people, we brought Harmony Hill into a place of really having a sense of itself.

"I am so deeply impressed and respectful of that staff and Gretchen, those who have been there for years, who have been open to learning and growing and agonizing and struggling; they're doing an amazing job as a professional organization."

During that time of "growing pains" at Harmony Hill, Lu was also experiencing her own personal struggle about who she was and what she was meant to do in the world because she had retired from her career.

"For me, that meant a journey back for another master's degree and some real inner-self exploration. For Harmony Hill, it was getting clear about what their mission is, about making the cancer retreats the center of everything they did.

"It was kind of like we were in our teenage years then, both Harmony Hill and I, struggling for identity and yet wanting to grow and move on and be more out in the world."

The year 2004 was an especially stressful one for the Farbers, who, since the previous year, had been caretakers for several friends and family members. Stu's mother died in February 2004, Stu was diagnosed with prostate cancer in June, and Lu's elderly parents moved in with them in October. In November 2004, Stu went in for surgery.

"When I decided to have surgery, what became clear to me was there was this medical side that I knew very well, but what I didn't know was how to prepare the other parts of me. On the personal level, cancer is a very intense opportunity to learn a lot about yourself.

"Gretchen was very helpful in terms of her counsel. It was my first introduction to meditation tapes and I found them very useful; I normally wouldn't do that kind of stuff. I also found yoga very helpful, and I just tried to center myself in the love and joy and peace of my life rather than be very fearful and anxious. Somehow or other I managed to show up that morning and they did the surgery and I survived."

Stu and Lu then attended a one-day cancer workshop at Harmony Hill.

"Harmony Hill was very supportive and helped enrich my experience – both through my personal connections with many of the practitioners who are a part of the program, and the workshop itself."

Reflecting on what effect his personal experience with cancer has had on his professional life, Stu says, "I was a doctor for 20 years in North Tacoma, and I delivered and took care of children. After I had become a parent I remember one of the mothers saying, 'Well, you know, you were always a pretty nice guy but now you *really* understand.' And I would say it's the same issue. Some of the highest praise in my work as a physician will be from people as I'm listening to them and trying to help them figure out the right thing for their medical needs, and occasionally an insightful person will say, 'You've had cancer, haven't you?' And they know that not because I do self-revelation, but they know that because of how I'm present and how I understand what they're going through. It's quite high praise because it's *the connection between us* that communicates that, not me saying, 'You think you have problems. When I had your problem, this is what I did.'

"So I would say on many levels it's made me much more empathic and understanding. Certainly my endorsement of alternative therapies is a lot stronger now. And even more than before, I'm very happy with myself and my life."

After his surgery, Stu got back to work at the end of January 2005. Then, in February, Lu was diagnosed with uterine cancer. She had her surgery in March.

"I just didn't have time to mess around with it; there was too much going on," she says. "Stu's recovery was very lengthy, and I had a lot of other people to take care of, so I went in for surgery and I was done. There were moments of fear, obviously, but my doctor said if you're going to have cancer, this is the best one to have, particularly if it's caught early.

"I used a lot of the suggestions that were offered, but we didn't actually go to a cancer retreat. I'd been there with Stu, and I'd been there with Gretchen in early 2002 as she was going through her cancer. But mostly, for me, it was 'Get it out, get it over with, get back to work,' because there were people who needed me."

A few years later, it was time for another transition: after seven years of serving on Harmony Hill's Board of Directors, it became clear to Lu that it was time for her to step off the Board.

"I felt like I had really given and done all that I could do. So I stepped away for several years, though of course I've always remained a friend to the Hill and to Gretchen.

"But I just got re-involved last year as faculty, and it feels very right to me because of my own journey. This is something I've thought about and talked about doing for many, many years. I'm very passionate about a movement technique called InterPlay, a way of accessing body wisdom, of becoming aware of what we're holding, and expressing and releasing it. Now I'm doing cancer retreats and helping to develop a Harmony Hill grief and loss retreat for people dealing with whatever kinds of grief and loss they face in their lives."

When asked to sum up what Harmony Hill means to him, without a moment's hesitation, Stu replies, "Peace and love.

"When Nordstrom Hall was completed, our son and his wife had just married. We had a reception there of our community, and we christened the Great Hall with its first event. It was a celebration of community and love, joy and peace, of all the generations. Every time I walk into that hall, I feel that connection."

"That's how connected we feel to the Hill," Lu agrees, "and the feeling is mutual. They're like family." ❖

> "Life is known only by those who have found a way to be comfortable with change and the unknown. Given the nature of life, there may be no security, only adventure."
>
> – RACHEL NAOMI REMEN

TRUEDA GOODING:
ONE DAY AT A TIME

Trueda Gooding's son, Joshua, was 25 years old and in graduate school when he was diagnosed with a malignant brain tumor. He was given a prognosis of two to five years. Trueda became his primary caregiver, at first from a distance as Josh tried to stay in school In California, and later more directly, when he moved back home. Through countless rounds of chemotherapy, she has been at his side, watching him on a roller-coaster of rallies and declines, both physical and cognitive. She has tried hard to balance his need for care and advocacy with his need to remain independent and autonomous as long as possible.

"He deserves to be treated as the adult that he is," she says.

One of the most painful and frightening aspects, for both Trueda and her son, is that "Joshua no longer gets my jokes. We always shared the same dry and somewhat twisted sense of humor. How I miss that!"

Living with Josh's illness has taught Trueda to take each day at a time and to live it fully, savoring the bloom of the cherry tree or the warmth of the sun on a crisp February day. She has learned to ask herself frequently, "What is there about this moment that I can find joy in?"

But caring for Josh for so many months also made Trueda hyper-vigilant.

"I was alert and 'on-duty' 24 hours a day. There was no down-time and I couldn't turn it off, no matter how hard I tried. I was bone-tired."

Trueda signed up for Harmony Hill's Caregivers Conference in May of 2009.

"I didn't go with huge expectations, but I knew I needed to get away. I was losing myself. I was getting grumpy in my interactions with others and showing a lot of the signs of burnout.

"The time off I had for those three days at Harmony Hill allowed me to break that vigilant behavior. I connected with other people. I connected with myself. It was like honey to my soul. I realized without knowing exactly how it happened that I was relaxed, and since leaving Harmony Hill I have been able to remain in touch with that relaxation. If I see myself starting to approach that hyper-alert state, I can control it. I can choose what I need to be for the situation or circumstance that presents itself."

Trueda is aware now that she can't keep going on unless she takes care of herself with as much love and kindness as she gives to others. She is committed to taking each day as it comes and living it fully.

"I realized that if we just keep putting one foot in front of the other, we will come out on the other side."

Another gift Trueda received from Harmony Hill was the opportunity to be with other caregivers, other people who understood what she was going through.

"I needed to be able to voice those things that I was feeling that I couldn't say in front of my family or friends, and know that there were others who sometimes felt the same. It eased the caregiver loneliness.

"Harmony Hill's setting was incredibly healing. I didn't have the energy for all of the activities, but just to be able to sit and drink in the view of the Hood Canal and the mountains was the most healing thing imaginable. It renewed me."

"There is so much more to life than what we see or understand. Harmony Hill was, for me, a catalyst for remembering myself and remembering that my job is to live to the fullest no matter what. Harmony Hill gave me a new beginning." ❖

"The more still, more patient and more open we are when we are sad, so much the deeper and so much the more unswervingly does the new go into us, so much better do we make it ours, so much the more will it be our destiny."

– RAINIER MARIA RILKE

GRETCHEN:
WE ARE FAMILY...

For many people, myself included, the concepts of "home" and "family" are closely related. Coming to Harmony Hill does feel like coming home, whether one is coming for the first time or the hundredth. I feel it every single time I drive up the hill and see the gardens that have provided beauty and nourishment to so many, and see the sturdy buildings that have offered comfort and safety to thousands. There is a sense of welcoming that can only be felt – words could never adequately describe it.

At the same time, coming home is more than just this extraordinary place. It's also the people – the Harmony Hill family. It's a big family, and it's constantly growing. As one of our staffers put it as she prepared to leave for a long-sought opportunity: *"I am deeply grateful for the gift I have been given in working here with all of you over the past few years. Harmony Hill has become a place I think of as another home – with all of you as my second family. Each one of you has touched my life in one way or another – and I am a better person because of it. This place and all of you will always have a special place in my heart wherever I go."*

The Harmony Hill family extends beyond staff. It encompasses our Board of Directors, our volunteers, donors, and neighbors. Just as each family is composed of individuals with disparate interests, skills, and temperaments that combine to create a unique whole, I often marvel at the distinctive skills, strengths, and heart-centered capacities that our staff and volunteers possess. The common thread is a passion for the work we do and the genuine and profound grace with which they serve.

We absolutely consider our retreat participants to be part of the clan. When we complete a cancer program I always tell them they are now part of the Harmony Hill family, and we want them to stay in touch, keep us posted on how they are doing, and come back – whether for more programs, or simply to enjoy the peace of the Hill. ❖

> "All growth is a leap in the dark, a spontaneous, unpremeditated act without the benefit of experience."
>
> – HENRY MILLER

ROSEMARY SPYHALSKY:
FINDING HER PLACE

Rosemary Spyhalsky, an oncology and chemotherapy nurse, first heard about Harmony Hill from one of her patients. She called the Hill to learn more and subsequently was invited to attend a half-day workshop for health professionals. The experience turned out to be life-changing.

"As soon as I arrived, I felt so welcome, so *seen*, it was like I belonged there. I didn't know anyone there, but we connected immediately and we shared our experiences and our struggles."

Melissa West led the group through a meditation to open the heart.

"It brought me to tears. Everything about that day was about opening the heart, and I just can't express how momentous that was. Everything shifted for me in just that half-day among people I had never met before. It's strange to say, but I felt like I had come home.

"At the time I came to the retreat, I was feeling a bit of a personal crisis in my own workplace. I was questioning what I was doing as a nurse, and whether working in oncology and chemotherapy was the right fit for me. I wondered: where were *my* heart and spirit in my nursing practice? Through this profound heart-opening experience I started to see that I had options; I realized that I could open up to exploring other ways to practice nursing in which I could still care for patients. Specifically, there was more that I could do to help people with cancer.

"As a chemotherapy nurse, I was so focused on how to help patients through the daunting experience of their treatment, but I didn't see the whole picture. It wasn't until I became a housemother at Harmony Hill that I could see some of the other challenges patients and their loved ones were facing. I became aware of holistic nursing, and the possibility of integrating body, mind, and spirit care. My nursing practice changed immensely during this time."

That half-day retreat was so moving Rosemary knew she wanted to come back for more. She volunteered to be a house mother for cancer retreats. She found each one to be a rich and powerful experience and learned so much listening to the stories participants told – stories about diagnosis, treatment, living with cancer, or caring for a partner who was dealing with cancer.

"It helped me to be a better nurse. Gretchen became my mentor and coach. She took me under her wing and introduced me to holistic nursing practice."

Rosemary particularly remembers an all-women's retreat she participated in: "Since it was for women only, most attendees were not with their partner or regular caregiver. They were women coming from separate lives, and they had to bond with one another in a different way. I remember one woman in particular who came very reluctantly and informed us that she probably would not stay. She came to Harmony Hill terrified of leaving her familiar life and spending a weekend with strangers, facing her diagnosis and talking about cancer. Something magical happened. She connected deeply with the group and realized that she wasn't alone in her experience or in her feelings. There was a huge shift; she saw everything differently. By the end of the weekend she didn't want to go home! I have heard Gretchen say many times during a retreat that the right people show up at the right time; I have witnessed this to be true time and time again at the cancer retreats."

At the same time she was volunteering at Harmony Hill, Rosemary enrolled in a holistic nursing education program, and took a leading role in developing an integrated cancer care program in the Providence Health System in Olympia. She also became a founding member of VOICE for Healing in Healthcare, a program committed to helping nurses discover and renew the heart and spirit of their work.

She is now working toward becoming a Nurse Practitioner with a Masters in nursing, and works as Nurse Coordinator at Providence Integrative Cancer Care. The growing program offers a variety of complementary therapies – including massage, yoga, acupuncture, nutrition, naturopathy – to patients undergoing conventional cancer treatment.

"There are many amazing providers here in the Olympia area. We help patients get the care they need – truly comprehensive care – in their own backyards. It's been a real learning process and bridge-building opportunity between the medical community and complementary providers."

Whenever possible, Rosemary encourages people to go to Harmony Hill, whether they are health professionals or individuals facing cancer.

"I feel so fortunate to have found Harmony Hill. It definitely transformed my life. The fact that there's no charge for the retreats makes them accessible to everyone. So many people wouldn't be able to go if they had to pay. It's wonderful that this life-changing experience is open to anyone." ❖

JOAN BREKKE:
DRAWN TO PEACE AND BEAUTY

When Joanie Brekke retired from Boeing, her friend Phyllis Woods said, "I think it's time for you to get acquainted with Harmony Hill."

While they had worked together at Boeing, Phyllis had told Joanie a lot about this organization, where she had done some pro bono work.

"She talked about it with such enthusiasm. I was interested," Joanie recalls, "so we arranged a time and she met me over there, at Harmony Hill. It was a gorgeous day in 2004, I believe; Gretchen was there, and Susan Keith, too.

"Right over lunch, sitting in that wonderful dining room, looking out over the Sound, they started talking about me being on the Board, and I said what I was really interested in was life-coaching the staff. They said you can do both! I said I didn't know about that, but I'd give it a try.

"At first, I thought, 'Why am I on this board?' All these statistics and finances made my head spin."

When she realized all those figures and financial data really came down to "people stuff," Joanie says, "I felt I could make a contribution there.

"I always said if there was a conflict between coaching staff members and my board duties, I would choose coaching. But there never was a conflict. I guess my role on the Board has changed a bit. For one thing, I've become more active in fundraising. I always said, 'Just don't ask me to fundraise: I can do anything but fundraise.' But that's not true."

In 2010, with rookie Joanie co-chairing the fundraising committee, close to $40,000 was raised for the Hill. Anyone who knows Joanie knows that whenever she puts her mind to something, she makes it happen.

"I feel that it's an honor – and that's how I've always felt – to be able to contribute to this organization. When it comes to the coaching, I get more out of it than anyone else, and it's the same thing working and helping with Harmony Hill: I get more out of it than they do.

"Harmony Hill touches me in my heart. Just being there, I feel different. The kind of work they do there is so phenomenal, it just makes me feel like I'm making a contribution in a way that feels very, very good. I think I appreciate life a little bit more than I did before. I appreciate health.

"And the people who work there are so extraordinary. I didn't know people could be as good as these people who are on staff at Harmony Hill. And Gretchen is fantastic; there's no one else like her. I have nothing but deep, deep respect for her."

Above all, it is the land – the Hill itself – that draws Joanie back again and again.

Her eyes light up as she talks about being on the grounds of Harmony Hill.

"My first time there, looking out on the flowers and the mountains and the water, when they asked me to participate, there was not a hesitation in my body because I had fallen in love. And that is the feeling I have every time I go back. There's a peacefulness and serenity that I haven't felt any other place. And it's always reoccurring; it's always there. When I'm on those grounds, something changes inside me. I understand how people get healed there. It's the place, it *is* the place.

"I can never imagine what it would be like to have cancer because I've never had it. But just to *be* there, to be close to nature, close to the earth, I think that a person would be able to relax in a different way and experience something that could profoundly change them. Even if it didn't profoundly change them, some type of healing would take place. Because even as a cancer-free person, you can't be there without feeling better. So if you have cancer, and are able to go through the program and the discussions and the whole thing, to me, it would be like somebody taking your body and putting it in their hands and saying to you, 'Now for two or three days I'm going to take care of you. You can let go.'

"Gretchen has made a believer of me. She always says the right people show up at the right time. And I've seen it, they do show up. Again and again and again. That's why it's going to grow and to thrive. *It's a healthy place that takes care of sick people.* And the people who are drawn to the place are the people to whom, just as it spoke to me, it will speak to them. Harmony Hill will continue to thrive because it's just meant to be." ❧

❝And the day came when the risk to remain tight in a bud was more painful than the risk it took to blossom."

– ANAÏS NIN

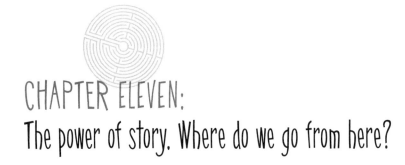

CHAPTER ELEVEN:
The power of story. Where do we go from here?

"I love how swiftly people enter into the intimacy of their personal stories, how there is a deep reverence for each person as they move through their challenges, and how the participants bond with each other with such natural ease. They ... move into their pain and fears, becoming more available and open to life." – CHRIS ADAMS, MD, CANCER RETREAT FACILITATOR

Throughout this book, stories have been shared – stories of people whose lives were touched by Harmony Hill and people who influenced the growth and direction of the Hill; people who remain active supporters of the Hill, and people who have departed this life, but whose spirits remain in our memories....

There is enormous power in story, whether it's the strength to tell our stories to strangers, the insights we gain from listening to the stories people share with us, or the awareness that in the telling of our stories we change, and so – miraculously – do our stories.

Story is one of the foundations of Harmony Hill – alongside caring staff and volunteers, nutritious and delicious food, a breathtaking natural setting, a safe and healing space, and deep and powerful connections.

There are so many ways of connecting with our stories. We can shout them from the roof-tops or we can whisper them to the night stars. We can tell them, write them, paint them, we can even *dance* our stories. The important thing is that we take the time to explore our stories either alone or with others. In the exploration and the interpretation, we create our reality, we define our experiences.

In Chapter Five, we met Ricardo Gomez, who started blogging as a way of keeping family and friends informed of his wife Claudia's progress through her cancer journey. Originally seen as a way of managing many calls, visits, and e-mails, it became, as Ricardo describes it, "my sacred space: it became my therapy and my window of conversation with friends, real or imagined." Writing gave Ricardo "the illusion of conversation" with loved ones spread far and wide, and it comforted him as he faced his fears and endeavored to remain strong for his family. "I write when my heart is ready to write, and it pours out."

Following Claudia's death, Ricardo continued to blog, to make sense of his grief, to sustain a feeling of connection, and ultimately to begin dealing with his own cancer diagnosis. He notes how the blog "has shaped and transformed everything, how it brings you all into my living room all the time...."

For Ricardo, writing in his blog (now a book) was how he connected to his story and how he made sense of it.

For Julie Barrett Ziegler, whom we met in Chapter Three, the way she understood and transformed her story was through her art. She refused to be defined by her diagnosis or by dehumanizing medical treatments. Through her art, she rediscovered her Self and renewed her purpose. She substituted the drab story others were writing for her with her own glorious and vivid story.

Time and again we've seen that words have power. Am I a cancer *victim* or a cancer *survivor*? Does "surrender" mean *giving up* or does it mean shifting one's perspective and *opening up* to new possibilities? Likewise, there is a world of difference between *losing control* and *releasing control*.

When we tell our stories, paying attention to the words we use and the ways our bodies react to them as we say them or think them, we can direct our stories to reveal our strength and our power.

> **"**In the silence of listening, you can know yourself in everyone, the unseen singing softly to itself and to you."
>
> – RACHEL NAOMI REMEN

We heard repeatedly from cancer survivors who realized that they may not have control over their diagnosis or even their prognosis, but they had control over their response to it, and *that* fact changed the world for them, and often for the people around them. We saw that what we choose to give our attention to and what we choose to tell when we tell our stories tells us who we are. There is such power in knowing that we can change anything by changing our attitude toward it. ❧

PAM REHWALD:
THE COMEBACK KID

Pam Rehwald is a vibrant woman with a glow that emanates from within. Twice diagnosed with a brain tumor and given a poor prognosis, twice Pam is a long-term survivor.

"I guess He's not ready for me yet – there's still more I have to do here. There's a reason I've been blessed."

Pam faced her first brain tumor in 1983, when she was a busy working mother of four, a wife, and a successful artist. That tumor – though not malignant – was inoperable, so she was treated with maximum doses of radiation. To the wonder of her medical team, she recovered fully – all except her hair, which never grew back in the irradiated area of her scalp. Then, in 1994, another brain tumor – this time malignant – was discovered and Pam's doctor told her there was "no hope."

"I'm feisty. I wasn't going to take that kind of talk. I changed doctors."

The second doctor wasn't so negative. He said if Pam was up for it, he would operate, but she must understand that there would be significant damage as a result. He performed a nine-hour surgery on Pam, removing one-quarter of her brain, including parts that govern speech, memory, and motor control. Pam emerged unable to do most of the tasks we take for granted.

"I had to relearn how to walk and talk, and how to read and write. They told me I'd better get used to using a wheelchair, but my dad was in a wheelchair for 25 years and I wasn't having any of that."

After one day, Pam tossed the wheelchair aside. And a few days later, she jettisoned the walker they had given her in its place. Is it any wonder that many have called Pam "The Comeback Kid"?

Today, 16 years later, Pam still has some mobility impairment, and words don't always come as easily as they once did, but Pam is undaunted: "This is the way I am. My limitations don't define me. I love life, I love people – I don't need to be any more than what I am."

What Pam is is authentic. She dresses with her own flair and always looks stylish. She's still an artist, too – painting, drawing, fabric arts. At one time, she even designed and built furniture.

"I'm slower than I used to be, but if I put a brush or a pencil in my hand, magic happens."

Her paintings are luminous, evoking scenes the viewer wants to step into. They reflect her inner and her outer worlds; they convey her soul. Pam sees the world with an artist's eye – appreciating the color and variety of her surroundings, just as she appreciates the color and variety of the people around her.

She has a gift for connecting with people – even perfect strangers – and she delights in kindness.

"Giving back is important to me. None of us is too busy for a kind word, or a smile. It takes so little to be nice to another human being, and it *always* comes back *to us*."

Pam attended a Harmony Hill cancer retreat in the late 1990s, while still rehabbing from her surgery. She recalls, "Everyone there was so wonderful to talk to. Each and every one of us had a story all our own, and each of us shared. Some were quieter and didn't say as much, and some were boisterous and loud. There were big stories and little stories, but each was unique, and each was straight from the heart. It meant so much to us to share our stories and to listen to each other's stories. I'll never forget that."

Pam especially remembers walking the labyrinth at Harmony Hill: "I still needed help with a lot of things at that time, but I wanted to walk the labyrinth alone. I went by myself, at my own speed, and it was magical! I felt so alive, and I also had this feeling that I could do anything ... I was a big girl now!" she laughs. "I've kept that feeling."

Faith has always been an important part of Pam's life. No matter what challenges were put in front of her, she always felt she would meet them and beat them.

"I never felt that I was alone, there was always someone beside me, helping me make it through. I'm here because I'm supposed to be here – there is a purpose – I believe that."

Pam would love to return to Harmony Hill for another retreat and another opportunity to walk the labyrinth.

"Coming to Harmony Hill felt like coming home. It's a place to go and feel safe." ❖

> " Three things in human life are important. The first is to be kind; the second is to be kind; and the third is to be kind."
>
> – HENRY JAMES

Each of us is on our own unique path. Whether we are facing a cancer diagnosis, caring for a loved one with cancer, a health care professional, volunteer, or simply reading this book for the inspiration of the people and the place – each of us has a story and is a participant in the stories of others. There is such power in that, such privilege! The more aware we are of our own story and the ways we can touch other people's stories, the more alive our stories become, and the more alive we become, as well. ❖

MARJORIE LUCKEY:
LEARNING TO BE

Barbara Riefle introduced Marjorie Luckey to Harmony Hill. The New York physician first traveled to Harmony Hill in 2003, several months after Barbara's death. She wanted to give back to the community, in gratitude for the contributions it made to the quality of her friend's life, so she had volunteered to be a housemother for a three-day cancer retreat.

"I had a remarkable experience, seeing people come to the retreat feeling very much the way that I had felt during my own experience with colon cancer that my life had been taken over by the cancer, that everything I had been before had faded out of the picture. My identity had come down to this: I was only a person with cancer, someone undergoing chemotherapy, someone undergoing radiation treatment. The fear of it overtook my life for a while – the fear, the sickness, the physical symptoms, and the struggle of trying to take care of my family, who were also very frightened. I came out of it with what felt like a post-traumatic disorder. My life felt like it had been dumped upside down and emptied out."

At Harmony Hill, Marjorie saw people arrive in that state, some of them still sick and not feeling well. She recognized that, as it had been for her, their entire worlds had changed the moment they received their diagnoses.

"After just two and a half days, those people were walking out of the retreat in a very different state. Nothing had changed about their physical condition, nothing had changed about their cancer prognosis or the experience they'd had, but clearly there was a feeling of *life* and of having their feet under them again."

While she was serving as a housemother at the retreat, Marjorie had a life-changing experience.

One of the participants had a diagnosis of lung cancer, several different lung cancers, in fact; she had undergone several surgeries, and then another cancer had shown up. She was facing the possibility of having another part of her lung removed, which could leave her a pulmonary cripple – she would need oxygen, wouldn't be able to get around well, and would have much trouble breathing.

Marjorie recalls that, "She was understandably quite upset about it. I think she had just about decided not to go through with any more surgery, to let the cancer go. She and her daughter had come to the retreat together. During the course of the weekend, the woman made it very clear that she did not want any kind of 'therapy,' she didn't want to discuss what she should do or shouldn't do; she didn't want to talk about her diagnosis or her decision.

"At that point I really wasn't sure what I could do for her; I didn't feel like I had anything to offer her. But she was such a fascinating, wonderful woman. She had done amazing things in her life, she'd had the inner strength to raise her three or four kids alone in the wilds of Alaska. Though she hadn't had much of an education before, she went back to school and had become a nurse practitioner. I sat up with her, just listening to her story and being totally amazed by her as a person.

"During the course of that weekend, she got back in touch with the person who had lived that life, the person who had that type of resilience and strength. I think that in talking about what her life had been like before, she remembered what it was like to live her life, to *be* her. And that's what she walked out with. I never found out what decision she made about the surgery, but that wasn't the issue. The issue was that she walked back into her life, fully in touch with who she was – with a lot of gratitude and joy about her own inner strength. She got back in touch with that kernel of her that can't be destroyed by adversity or cancer or chemotherapy or even death – the essence of her Self. She walked away from that retreat with a kind of radiance – the radiance that I had heard in the life that she had lived."

To realize what truly happens to people who undergo cancer or any other great trauma was a profound revelation to Marjorie.

"The way our medical system deals with cancer and other serious disease is like being in a war. The focus of Western medicine, of which I am a part, is to focus on the disease and to figure out how to *fight* the disease. The thing that is missing is focusing on what is healthy, what brings more energy and life to the body. What happens at these retreat weekends is that people are able to get back to what is *healthy* about themselves.

"It's not easy to do that. It *sounds* easy on the surface – *'oh, well, now I'll just focus on what is healthy'* – but you've been in this battle with a very scary enemy and there's no guarantee that you're going to win. The weapons used can make you sick, drain your energy and set you up for infections, but they can also be effective and curative, so most people choose them. Under these circumstances, it can be hard to reconnect with who we really are, with what's healthy and good in our lives. That's easier to do in happier times but difficult to do when we're putting all of our energies into survival."

At the time of the retreat, Marjorie had been finished with her own cancer for about a year, though her doctors couldn't declare her cured until she'd gone five years without a recurrence.

"As a housemom, I felt like I received a tremendous amount of healing for myself, that I was able to reconnect to what was healthy and good in my own life. It's also been a great help when I've had to deal with other challenges. Since then, for example, I had a major femur fracture and a 'flesh-eating bacteria infection' developed in my foot. I was either in the hospital or in bed for three months, and what I learned at the retreat enabled me to stay more connected with all that was healthy. Despite the fear of losing my foot, I was able to say, 'My foot and my leg have a big problem, but the rest of me is fine' – and that was a way for me to stay in touch with what was most important in my life."

Her experience with Harmony Hill has had an effect on Marjorie's work as a physician, as well as her personal life.

"I recognized how I've been trained in Western medicine to focus on the disease. My Harmony Hill encounters have caused me to take a much bigger view of my patients' lives, particularly the ones who are having a very hard time with their diagnoses. Sometimes all it takes is spending time talking with them, with me not saying very much, allowing them to tell me about their lives. In the retelling of their lives, they seem to get more in touch with themselves – the parts that they love, the parts that reward them, the parts that give them joy. And they walk out of my office feeling their disease diminished, that it hasn't completely overtaken their lives."

Though she felt that the cancer retreat was amazingly successful for the participants, Marjorie found herself feeling guilty at the end of it. In talking it over with Gretchen afterward, Marjorie told her that she hadn't made any contribution there at all.

"My job, as I saw it, was to make tea for somebody who wasn't feeling well or, if somebody was upset, my job was to comfort them. But nobody in my house had any physical needs that I could fulfill, and no one was looking for comfort. I felt that I'd been pretty worthless as a housemom. Then Gretchen told me that the woman I'd listened to and her daughter had both mentioned that I had played a key role in her positive experience at Harmony Hill. I was totally baffled by that because I had done nothing, really and truly nothing, except to selfishly ask her to tell me more about her life because I found it and her so interesting.

"When Gretchen said to me, 'It was your *being*, not your *doing*, that helped that woman,' I didn't understand what she meant. All my life I have been a doer; my profession is *to do*: to diagnosis illness or to explain, to teach, to help people. So the concept – that I might *do* nothing and that somehow this characteristic of *being* would have an influence – baffled me. So I walked the labyrinth around *She Who Knows* with the question of "How does one *BE*? It kind of started an important journey for me, wherein I have come to realize that there is an essence, this quality in everyone; that if I was paralyzed or locked away in a cell, there would still *be* that something.

"The question about *being* which began for me that weekend at Harmony Hill is really a profound one. I know now that for my friends and family, who I am, how I listen, and the love I have for them are the things that are most important to them, not what I *do*. And I believe the same thing is true for my patients, as well. There are times when my being has been a lot more important to them than my doing. I know that my compassion for them and my listening to them has truly helped them to reconnect with their own essential being and strength." ❖

> "It is not the nature of the task, but its consecration, that is the vital thing."
>
> – MARTIN BUBER

Harmony Hill's story is only half-told. It is still unfolding. As we celebrate our 25th year, we're looking forward to new and expanded programs: more one-day and three-day cancer retreats, grief retreats – both the group retreats and customized retreats for individual families. We're inaugurating the SuperSibs! Program and getting involved in the Nightingale Initiative. We're continuing to offer classes in wellness, cooking, gardening, movement, and healthy living, and making the Hill available to outside groups and individuals for corporate or personal retreats. There will undoubtedly be other offerings and other opportunities. Over these 25 years, Harmony Hill has grown from an idea of possibilities to a remarkable home of healing and hope. It is exciting to think what the next 25 years may bring. ❖

Supersibs! Another step in Harmony Hill's evolution

My name is Hannah, and I'm 11 years old. My mom having cancer has been a huge problem in my life. I've lost so many tears, and had my heart ripped out of me so many times. My mom having cancer has been the hardest thing ever because she's my best friend.

My mom has had cancer most of my life. She's been fighting it for ten years. I really didn't have anyone to talk to and to share my story with, not even my mom because she was so sick.

I remember my mom's first visit to Harmony Hill. She had the most amazing time and I was so happy she could tell someone who understood what she went through – someone who had cancer, too. It got me thinking how nice it would be to be able to tell my story. So I told my mom about a brilliant idea. What if we had a retreat for kids who had to go through what I had to go through, and we would all be able to talk about it together? We wouldn't be afraid to tell our story to other children, because they'd understand.

Hannah was eight years old when she brought up her brilliant idea, and it was the springboard for Harmony Hill's plans to develop new programs for families, particularly children, whose lives are affected by cancer.

The first step in that direction was Harmony Hill's winning the competition for LIVESTRONG Foundation funding for the SuperSibs! program, focusing on teens who have a sibling living with cancer. This program will serve as the perfect blueprint for Hannah's original idea, with future retreats serving children, their parents and grandparents – because cancer is a family disease.

SuperSibs!: Beginning in 2011, Harmony Hill will offer three-day retreats to families who have a teenaged child and a child with cancer.

Each day **46** children are diagnosed with cancer. That's **12,500** children each year.

And for every one of these children newly-diagnosed with cancer, there is an extended family – dramatically multiplying the number of people affected by one child's disease. The numbers are staggering, and the emotional toll is enormous.

Parents are emotionally and physically drained as they struggle to attend the needs of their child with cancer, to deal with doctors' appointments, medical procedures and the myriad decisions that must be made.

Brothers and sisters of a child with cancer have been called cancer's "shadow survivors." Often these siblings feel insignificant, afraid and ignored, as their parents are simply unable to find the energy to be fully present for their healthy children's needs and attention. Under the best of circumstances, the teenage years can be emotionally tumultuous; given the stress and tremendous changes caused by cancer in the family, the shadow survivors' teenaged years can be devastating.

Due to the support of the LIVESTRONG SuperSibs! funding, these retreats are offered at no cost to participants. The program will focus on individual and family needs, provide stress reduction skills, guided imagery, and support groups. Teens will be able to enjoy a wide range of activities such as art, kayaking and other outdoor pursuits, as well as nutrition, movement, and self-care sessions.

The Harmony Hill SuperSibs! program is designed to give teens and their families a sense of renewal, a time to reconnect with themselves and with each other, and to provide them with the resources and ongoing support to sustain them through difficult times and beyond. ❖

"Deep listening is miraculous for both listener and speaker. When someone receives us with open-hearted, non-judging, intensely interested listening, our spirits expand."

– SUE PATTON THOELE

Harmony Hill's story has been unfolding for 25 years. Countless people have been part of that story, just as Harmony Hill and people encountered there have played parts in so many individuals' stories. The beauty and mystery of it all is that the stories go on forever and we'll never know where they will touch others, or how, or who. ❖

GRETCHEN:
AND THE STORIES GO ON...

It's been nearly ten years since my original diagnosis of Non-Hodgkin's Lymphoma, nearly five years since my recurrence. I have periodic CT scans to see if there has been another recurrence. The scans are always cause for some anxiety, and time slows to a painful crawl during the wait between the test and getting the test results. I don't think I'm alone in feeling reluctant to talk too much about these CT scans. I don't want my friends or family to become apprehensive; I don't want them to always feel on alert; and I don't want them to get tired of hearing about my cancer journey. I'm happy to report, though, that my latest CT scan was clear, with no cause for worry. I feel so blessed to live here, and to have the health and energy to be a part of Harmony Hill's ongoing growth and service.

After 25 years as executive director of this remarkable place, it's time for my role to change. I'm looking forward to focusing my attention on our external connections with the American Holistic Nurses Association, the Northwest Organization of Nurse Executives, the BirchTree Center for Health Care Transformation, and NIGH, the Nightingale Initiative on Global Health, as well our vision of the Hill taking on a new additional role as the Northwest Center for Nurse Renewal.

I anticipate working with the next executive director who will lead efforts to expand Harmony Hill's cancer retreats, caregiver retreats, grief retreats, and retreats for kids whose families are struggling with cancer. It will be my pleasure to continue working with the remarkable staff, Board, and volunteers who have given so much of their time and energy to grow this place to what it is today ... and will be tomorrow. And I am relishing the prospect of spending more time in the gardens on this glorious Hill with its majestic views of the Olympic Mountain range.

My story started in the shadow of a magnificent mountain, and mountains have been an important part of my life since my earliest years. I look forward to more mountains, and, especially, more stories – stories of Harmony Hill, and rich stories of hope, healing, and homecoming.

My heartfelt wish for each of us is that our stories help us connect with one another, and that through both the stories and the connections, we find meaning, wholeness, and delight.

Blessings and thanks to all who have touched Harmony Hill, and to all who will as the Hill continues to evolve. ❖

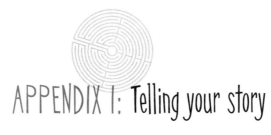

APPENDIX 1: Telling your story

"There is no greater agony than bearing an untold story inside of you."
— MAYA ANGELOU

What are your stories? The ones you tell others and the ones you tell yourself. Take some time to tell some of your stories. Tell them to family or friends, and take time to listen to theirs, as well. Or, if you prefer, tell your stories just to yourself. Sit in a quiet place and think about your stories or take a long walk and let your stories accompany you. Perhaps you'd prefer to write them down, or tell them through drawing, painting, or collage. Perhaps through movement or music – stories can be told in countless ways.

However you choose to tell your stories, don't direct them or judge them; allow them to unfold and simply be present for the unfolding. Don't be surprised if you start to see your life's experiences with new eyes.

If you're not sure how or where to start telling your stories, start with an experience and then with questions: What was happening in my life? What changed? What didn't? What images have stayed with me? Who am I as a result of my experience? What do I see now that I didn't see then? What do I see differently?

> **"**Stories differ from advice in that once you get them, they become a fabric of your soul That is why they heal you.**"**
> — ALICE WALKER

Hold your stories loosely. Allow your stories to surprise you. Allow them to make you laugh or make you cry. And allow them to change with distance and new insights you may have gained. Realize that your stories are never complete – as you grow and change, so do your stories. A story of pain and loss can transform into a story of wisdom and discovery. A story that we once perceived as describing our weakness can become the story of strength unfolding.

Embark on the adventure of a lifetime: start telling your stories...

There are countless resources that can either inspire or guide you as you begin telling your stories. Here are a few of our favorites:

Kitchen Table Wisdom, Rachel Naomi Remen, MD

My Grandfather's Blessings, Rachel Naomi Remen, MD

Storycatcher: Making Sense of Our Lives through the Power and Practice of Story, Christina Baldwin

Life's Companion: Journal Writing As a Spiritual Quest, Christina Baldwin

Lifelines: How Personal Writing Can Save Your Life, Christina Baldwin (set of 6 CDs)

Creative is a Verb: If You're Alive, You're Creative, Patty Digh

Inventing the Truth: The Art and Craft of Memoir, edited by William Zinsser

Legacy: A Step by Step Guide to Writing Personal History, Linda Spence

The Artist's Way, Julia Cameron

Writing Down the Bones, Natalie Goldberg

Listening is an Act of Love, edited by David Isay, StoryCorps

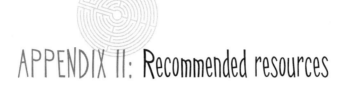

APPENDIX II: Recommended resources

Memoir, Inspiration, and Information

Last Adventure of Life, Maria Dancing Heart

It's Not About the Hair, Debra Jarvis

Chasing Daylight: How My Forthcoming Death Transformed My Life, Eugene O'Kelley

Kitchen Table Wisdom: Stories That Heal, Rachel Naomi Remen

My Grandfather's Blessings: Stories of Strength, Refuge, and Belonging, Rachel Naomi Remen

Conversations at Midnight: Coming to Terms with Dying and Death, Kay & Herbert Kramer

How to Go On Living When Someone You Love Dies, Therese Rando

How, Then, Shall We Live? Four Simple Questions That Reveal the Beauty and Meaning of Our Lives, Wayne Muller

It's Not About the Bike, Lance Armstrong

A Path with Heart, Jack Kornfield

When Things Fall Apart, Pema Chodron

The Places that Scare You, Pema Chodron

Crazy Sexy Cancer Tips, Kris Carr

Crazy Sexy Cancer Survivor: More Rebellion and Fire for Your Healing Journey, Kris Carr

Life is a Verb: 37 Days to Wake Up, Be Mindful, and Live Intentionally, Patty Digh

Glad No Matter What: Transforming Loss and Change into Gift and Opportunity, SARK

Close to the Bone: Life-Threatening Illness & the Search for Meaning, Jean Shinoda Bolen

The Book of Awakening, Mark Nepo

The Power of Now, Eckhart Tolle

Full Catastrophe Living, Jon Kabat-Zinn

Coming to Our Senses, Jon Kabat-Zinn

We Can Cope: Helping Parents Help Children When A Parent Has Cancer, Jonas Bromberg, Caroline McCabe, and Andrea Patenaude

Cancer Happens: Coming of Age with Cancer, Rebecca Gifford

Cancer Has Its Privileges: Stories of Hope and Laughter, Christine Clifford

Cancer Schmancer, Fran Drescher

Cancer Talk, Selma Schimmel and Barry Fox

Facing the Mirror with Cancer, Lori Ovitz

Exploring the Labyrinth: A Guide for Healing and Spiritual Growth, Melissa Gayle West

Silver Linings: The Power of Trauma to Transform Your Life, Melissa Gayle West

Healing Conversations: What to Say When You Don't Know What to Say, Nance Guilmartin

My Daddy's Cancer and *My Mommy's Cancer*, both by Cindy Cohen and John Heiney

Return to Wholeness: Embracing Body, Mind, and Spirit in the Face of Cancer, David Simon

Staying Well With Guided Imagery, Belleruth Naparstek

Health & Treatment

Cell-Level Healing: The Bridge from Soul to Cell, Joyce Hawkes

Fighting Cancer from Within, Mitchell Gaynor

Healing Essence: A Cancer Doctor's Practical Program for Hope and Recovery, Mitchell Gaynor

Choices in Healing: Integrating the Best of Conventional and Complementary Approaches to Cancer, Michael Lerner

Complementary Cancer Therapies, Dan Labriola

Coping With Lymphedema, Joan Swirsky and Diane Nannery

Journey Through Cancer: An Oncologist's Seven-Level Program for Healing and Transforming the Whole Person, Jeremy Geffen

Sexuality and Fertility after Cancer, Leslie Schover

Surgery: A Patient's Guide from Diagnosis to Recovery, Claire Mailhot, Melinda Brubaker, and Linda Slezak

Anticancer: A New Way of Life, David Servan-Schreiber, MD

Nutrition & Cookbooks

The Harmony Hill Cookbook

The Cancer Fighting Kitchen, Rebecca Katz

How to Prevent and Treat Cancer with Natural Medicine, Murray et al.

The China Study, T. Colin Campbell

What to Eat Now: The Cancer Lifeline Cookbook, Rachel Keim and Ginny Smith

The Cancer Prevention Diet, Michiko Kushi

Other Resources (Tapes, CDs, Websites)
Cancer in General

www.canceradvocacy.org/toolbox, on this site you'll find the Cancer Survival Toolbox(r), a free, self-learning audio program that has been developed by leading cancer organizations to help people develop important skills to better meet and understand the challenges of their illness

www.healthjourneys.com, guided imagery CDs by Belleruth Naparstek and others; many CDs specific to cancer, as well as other health issues, and general wellness

Gilda's Club, www.gildasclub.org, (888) 445-3248; provides social/emotional support, lectures, workshops, networking groups, and children's programs

American Cancer Society, www.cancer.org, (800) 227-2345

Susan G. Komen Foundation, www.komen.org, extensive resources for dealing with breast cancer

Caring Bridge, www.CaringBridge.com,offers free personalized Web sites to those wishing to stay in touch with family and friends during significant life events

Live Strong (Lance Armstrong's program), www.livestrong.org, survivorship topics and tools

MD Anderson Cancer Center, www.mdanderson.org, provides comprehensive information on research, clinical trials, prevention, support programs and related topics

CanHelp, www.canhelp.com, information about alternative cancer treatments including cutting edge and innovative therapies

Breast Cancer Mailing List, www.bclist.org, 24/7 online support group to give and receive support, share experiences

Chemo Care, www.chemocare.com, up-to-date information on chemotherapy

Mautner Project for Lesbians, www.mautnerproject.org, information and links for lesbians with cancer

www.lymphnet.org, education and guidance for lymphedema patients, as well as information on prevention of lymphedema

National Association of Breast Cancer Organizations, www.nabco.org, provides breast cancer information

www.cancerquest.org, biology of cancer and cancer treatments through award-winning graphics

National Ovarian Cancer Coalition, www.ovarian.org, information and resources for women with ovarian cancer

Oncolink, www.oncolink.com, treatment options, clinical trial information, resources

Mothers Supporting Daughters with Breast Cancer, www.mothersdaughters.org, helps women whose daughters have breast cancer

Pregnancy with Cancer, www.pregnantwithcancer.org, network of surviving women who had cancer while pregnant

Sisters Network National Headquarters, www.sisternetworkinc.org, African-American breast cancer survivors' organization

Healing Journeys, www.healingjourneys.com, free inspirational conferences for those touched by cancer

Support & Caregiver Resources

Share the Care, www.sharethecare.org, how to organize a group to care for someone who is seriously ill

Cancer and Careers, www.cancerandcareers.org, a resource for working women with cancer

Look Good...Feel Better, www.lookgoodfeelbetter.org, helps women manage changes in their appearance from cancer treatment

Living Beyond Breast Cancer, www.lbbc.org, a site oriented to survivors with news about conferences, special events, outreach programs, message boards

National Coalition for Cancer Survivorship, www.canceradvocacy.org, empowers survivors and advocates for policy issues that affect quality of life

Association of Online Resources, www.acor.org, offers access to mailing lists that provide support, information, and community to everyone affected by cancer and related disorders

Cancervive, www.cancervive.org, emotional support, information and advocacy

National Hospice and Palliative Care Organization, www.nhpco.org, can help you find answers to questions such as how to find hospice care, what to expect, and medical coverage for such care

Strength for Caring, www.strengthforcaring.com, an education and support website for cancer caregivers (including non-professionals) who provide care for loved ones with cancer

www.cancerclub.com, services and products to bring laughter to the lives of those with cancer and their caregivers

Young People

Young Survival Coalition, www.youngsurvival.org, group of survivors bringing people together to further issues surrounding breast cancer in young women

Planet Cancer, www.planetcancer.org, support for young adults with cancer

Group Loop, www.grouploop.org, website for teens with cancer, and their parents

The Ulman Cancer Fund for Young Adults, www.ulmanfund.org, support for young adults with cancer and their family and friends

Young People (continued)

KidsCope, www.kidscope.org, helps families and children understand the effects of cancer on a parent using educational material

Kids Konnected, www.kidskonnected.org, online support for kids who have a parent with cancer; good resource for parents

Financial and Legal Assistance

BenefitsCheckUp, www.benefitscheckup.org, locates programs for those 55+ years of age that will help pay for medical costs and services

CancerCare, www.cancercare.org, financial assistance and referrals

The Medicine Program, www.themedicineprogram.com, free prescription medicine nationwide

Medicare Information, www.medicare.gov, Federal insurance program of those 65+ years of age or those under 65 that are disabled

Patient Advocate Foundation, www.patientadvocate.org, provides education, legal counseling, and referrals concerning financial issues

Air Charity Network, www.aircharitynetwork.org, free nationwide service that flies patients to treatment centers nationwide

National Association of Hospital Hospitality Houses, (800) 542-9730, http://www.nahhh.org, guide to family-centered lodging and support services for families and their loved ones who are receiving medical treatment far from their homes

FertileHOPE, www.fertilehope.org, provides fertility preservation and financial assistance options for patients whose medical treatments threaten reproductive function

Corporate Angel Network, www.corpangelnetwork.org, free air transportation for cancer patients

Other

CancerGifts.com, www.cancergifts.com, gift baskets to provide hope, encouragement and comfort for people with cancer

Locks of Love, www.locksoflove.org, a public non-profit organization that provides hairpieces for financially disadvantaged children under age 18 suffering from long term medical hair loss from any diagnosis

Resources Local to Harmony Hill
(your community will likely have similar resources)

Harmony Hill Retreat Center, www.harmonyhill.org, (360) 898-2363; No-cost cancer retreats

Susan G. Komen Foundation, www.komenpugetsound.org, extensive resources for dealing with breast cancer

Providence Sound Home Care & Hospice, Shelton, WA, (800) 869-7062, support group to deal with grief reactions in daily life – no cost

Living for Today – Support Group, Belfair, WA, (360) 275-3714

Providence Integrative Cancer Care, Lacey, WA, (360) 412-8951; www.providence.org/southwest-washington/facilities/pmg/regional-cancer-center/integrative-cancer-care/; provides local resources for cancer patients and their families in Southwest Washington by addressing the mind, body, and spirit to improve quality of life

Breast Cancer Resource Center; Tacoma, WA (253) 753-4222, www.bcrcwa.org, free mammograms, library, wigs, prostheses, support groups, one-on-one peer support

Cancer LifeLine, www.cancerlifeline.org, provides information and support for people with cancer and their caregivers. Also provides support programs and classes for patients and families in the Seattle area. 24-hour lifeline, (800) 255-5505

Seattle Cancer Care Alliance, www.seattlecca.org, unites 3 internationally renowned cancer care institutions-Fred Hutchinson Cancer Research Center, UW Medicine, and Children's Hospital and Regional Medical Center-to offer a variety of treatment options, designed from the latest research, for malignant and non-malignant diseases

Sisters of Hope, Tacoma, WA, http://sistersofhopecancersupportgroup.org, (253) 572-2683, spiritual, emotional and sisterly support for women of color and others with cancer

Northwest Hope and Healing, www.northwesthopeandhealing.org, provides child care, transportation, meals, and education to women receiving breast cancer treatment

Team Survivor Northwest, www.teamsurvivornw.org, a group of supportive women bound by the common experience of a cancer diagnosis and an interest in living fit, healthy, active lifestyles

Community Health Education, Swedish Cancer Institute (206) 386-2502; free classes for anyone with cancer (not just Swedish patients)

Kitsap Cancer Services - Humble Abode, providing life enhancing support services for cancer patients, family, friends & caregivers, www.kitsapcancerservices.org

(If you've found other resources helpful on your journey, please share them with us. E-mail your suggestions to info@harmonyhill.org.)

APPENDIX III: Harmony Hill timeline

1985
- Gretchen attends retreat at St. Andrews House
- $700 received from Thurston-Mason County Social Services for Mason Co. Drug & Alcohol Abuse Prevention (MCDAP) program

1986
- Gretchen moves in as caretaker
- Board of Directors established
- Nonprofit incorporation granted
- Initial name "Harmony House"

1987
- Mission refined
- Greenhouse built with donated materials
- Garden restoration begins
- Gretchen joins local Volunteer Fire Dept (#622)

1988-1999
- Kitty & Elmer Nordstrom buy property
- 501(c)(3) Charitable status granted by IRS
- Lodge improvements begin

1990
- Name changed to Harmony Hill
- 10-year lease signed
- First Wellness Festival

1991-1992
- Wellness Programs begin
- Fiercely Independent Elders (FIEs) begin meeting
- First cookbook published

1993
- Training received at Commonweal
- Kitchen renovation and dining room expansion
- Crews from Purdy Women's Correctional Center begin working
- 1.5 Full time equivalent employees (FTEs)

1994
- First Cancer Program offered, named Fully Alive Retreat
- Garden labyrinth completed and garden expanded
- Guest Cottage added expands accommodations to 16

1995
- 15-year lease + 25-year renewal option signed
- Cancer Program: 29 participants

1996-1997
- Website developed
- Cancer Program: 60 served in 7 programs
- Sequoia Tree Labyrinth completed
- Business plan developed
- Yurt added
- 3 FTEs

1998
- 19 people attend 3 Cancer Retreats
- Bill & Melinda Gates Foundation provides major funding
- Database upgraded, accounting system purchased
- 5 FTEs

1999
- 37 attend cancer retreats
- Alliances with MultiCare, Cancer Lifeline and Commonweal
- Boeing funds allow for upgrades to communication system
- 40-year lease signed

2000
- Outreach to Health Professionals begins
- 60 participants in Cancer Retreats
- Seattle Foundation funds improvements
- Cheney funds Resource Center and Library
- NY Marathon fundraiser begins
- Gathering of Hearts to honor Kitty Nordstrom

2001
- Program expansion via Gates funding
- 71 attend Cancer Retreats
- First new building (office, shop, and apartment) and lavender labyrinth completed
- New septic system installed, Lodge upgraded
- 8.2 FTEs

2002
- Health Professional and Spa for the Soul programs begin
- Annex remodeled, modular office purchased
- 66 attend Cancer Retreats
- 12 FTEs

2003
- 88 attend Cancer Program
- First Offsite workshops conducted
- Boeing funds ADA and storm water runoff project, Simpson funds well and septic upgrade
- 11.7 FTEs

2004
- Cancer Program offered at no cost
- 139 attend Cancer Program, wait-list established
- Tools for the Journey one-day workshop started
- Kitchen upgraded to commercial status
- Seattle Foundation capital grant allows for construction of new guest lodge
- Major Gift Campaign begins
- 12 FTEs

2005
- 262 served in Cancer Program
- Thriving Beyond Cancer 1-day program started
- Creekside Lodge completed, overnight capacity expands from 16 to 30
- HG Runnings Conference Room dedicated at SummerFest
- 15.2 FTEs

2006

- 297 served in Cancer Program
- Elmer and Katharine Nordstrom Great Hall completed
- 1st Anna's Bay Music Festival concert held
- New 20th Anniversary Cookbook published
- Susan Russell Hall Paintings donated
- Bill & Melinda Gates Foundation Challenge Grant begins
- 15 FTEs

2007

- 267 served in Cancer Program
- DVD created by Christopher Davenport of 501 Productions
- New logo crafted by Howard Leggett
- "In Harmony" Program added
- Weekday Yoga added
- New garden labyrinth constructed
- 15.3 FTEs

2008

- 355 served in Cancer Program
- Collaborations with Multicare, UW-Tacoma, TAM to bring Lynne Twist to Northwest
- Lynne Twist: Soul of Money program at Harmony HIll
- Bill & Melinda Gates Foundation Challenge Grant reaches goal!
- 15.4 FTEs

2009

- 331 served in Cancer Program
- Deconstruction of Annex building
- Gate House under construction
- Ta'i Ji with Chung Liang started
- Wellness Program offerings expanded
- 15 FTEs

2010

- 421 served in Cancer Program
- First group of "triple" Extended Cancer Retreats (3 groups of 9)
- First Annual Survivorship Fair attended by 100
- Nurse Renewal Programs begin
- Lifestyle Change for Women Programs begin
- 24'x26' Greenhouse donated by Boeing Employees
- New "GateHouse" complete, accommodations now at 35 beds,
- Four tent sites constructed with lighted trail to Great Hall bathrooms
- Next decade visioning workshops held at Harmony Hill
- 15.3 FTEs

2011

- 25th Anniversary year!
- 425 projected to be served in Cancer Program
- All Cancer Program retreats now "triples" except Grief & Loss
- 2nd Annual Survivorship Fair in September
- SuperSibs program begins for teens/ families
- Inauguration of the Northwest Center for Nurse Renewal
- Yoga three times weekly open to community
- July/August rentals largest in our history
- *One Hill, Many Voices: Stories of Hope and Healing* is published
- Search for new Executive Director begins as Gretchen assumes a new role
- 14 FTEs

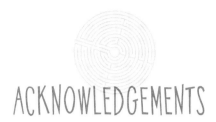

ACKNOWLEDGEMENTS

So many lights illuminated our path as we wrote this book, and to each we are eternally grateful.

Foremost among them is the radiant Gretchen Schodde, whose vision, energy and kind spirit infused our work, as it has infused Harmony Hill for 25 years. She connected us with the people we interviewed and spent hours telling "The Dragon" (making recordings of) her own life story.

Each of the individuals we spoke with – who told their own story or helped us to tell another's story – gave us the gift of their precious time, their hard-won wisdom, and their generosity of spirit. We enjoyed every conversation immensely and we learned so much from them.

For their careful reading and valuable suggestions, we thank Paul Leathers and Mary Ann Fraser.

We are indebted to Holly Harmon for her graphic design talent, her enthusiasm, commitment, great suggestions and good humor. Cheers to Kathleen Bauknight for recommending her to us.

For the wonderful images throughout the book, we are thankful to photographers Victrinia Ridgeway, Rodika Tollefson, Carolyn McIntyre, and Fatema Bannazadeh.

To the Board, staff and volunteers of Harmony Hill: the community you have created through your dedication and commitment is unlike any other and testament to your compassion and imagination.

We especially appreciate the Board and staff members who have been so helpful and heartening; for listening to and engaging in endless discussions over the past two years about this project, despite your own extensive workloads.

Many thanks to the FOBs, FIEs, VOICE nurses, housemoms, Jolene Black, Ann Lovejoy, the talented folks at Gorham Printing, and the many, many supporters of Harmony Hill whose generosity keeps the light shining ever so brightly.

And to our husbands, Paul Leathers and Bill Wiederkehr, whose patience, encouragement, support, and good humor were always with us.

Our thanks and blessing to each of you. ❖

(D.C. and K.L.)

ABOUT THE AUTHORS

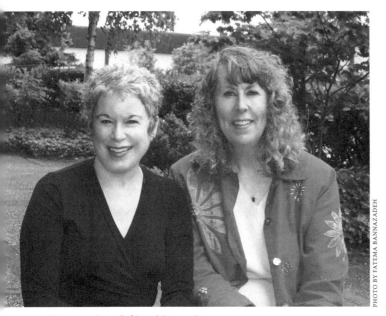

Kristen Leathers (left) and Donna Cameron.

Donna Cameron is a writer, speaker, and consultant. She is President of Melby, Cameron & Anderson, a Seattle-area company that works with non-profit organizations and associations. Donna has had numerous articles published in business, trade and professional publications. A firm believer in the power of story to heal and change lives, she lives in Brier, Washington, with her husband, Bill Wiederkehr.

Kristen Leathers is a freelance writer and editor. Since earning her MFA at Eastern Washington University, she's taught English, literature, and creative writing at Spokane Falls Community College and EWU, as well as private and nonprofit workshops. Her short stories, nonfiction articles and essays have been published in numerous magazines, newspapers, and literary journals, including *Willow Springs* and *Glimmer Train*. Currently, she serves on the Board of Directors at Harmony Hill and resides in Bellevue, Washington, with her husband Paul. ❧